SMOKE AND MIRRORS:

Echoes From an Iron Lung

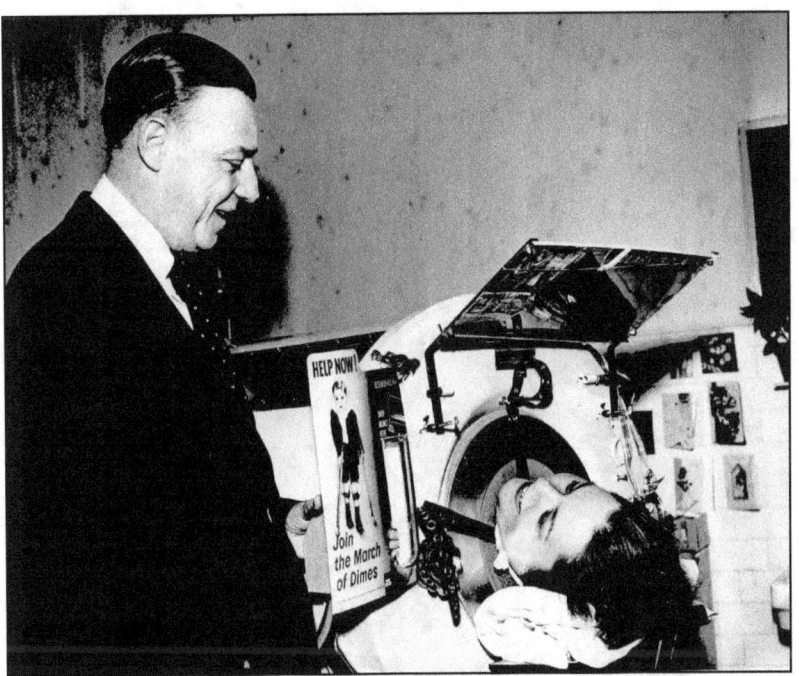

Christopher M. Clarke
and
Lorraine Reynolds Woodruff Clarke

For Mom

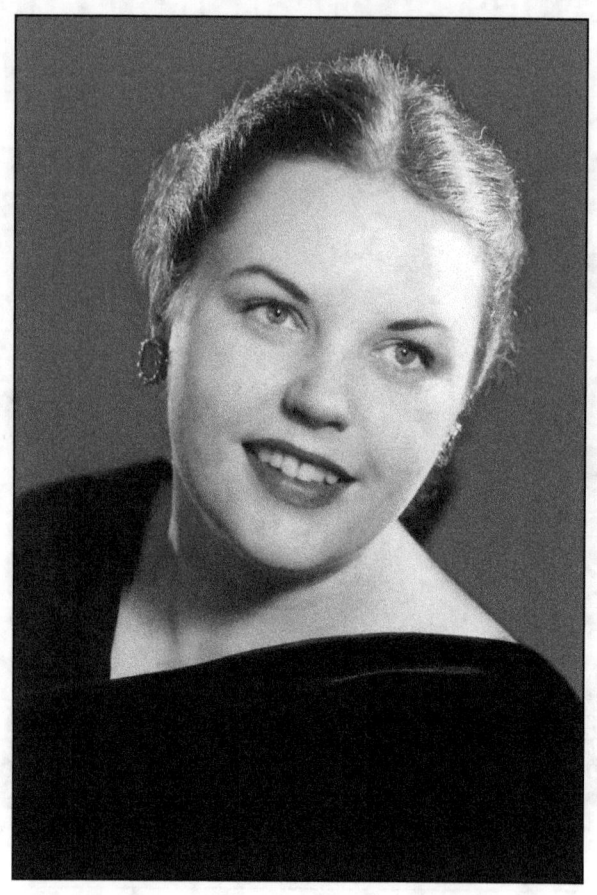

Clarke's Canyon Publishing
Huntingtown, Maryland

UNTITLED

I mean to cling to life as long as it will have me.
And whether that be
long or short,
then or now,
here or there,
who can tell?
Who can gainsay the future?
Only this do I know full well:
That where-so-ever you may be,
even the essence of you,
there shall I make my way also;
if I must batter down the very gates of Heaven
or plumb the utmost depths of Hell.

Rainie Clarke (1920-1965)

Preface

Life's not fair. If you don't believe me, just ask my mother, Lorraine Reynolds Woodruff Clarke ("Rainie"). But, wait! You can't. She died at 44 when I was barely 16. That's not fair.

Fair or not, Rainie never complained. Few have faced as many obstacles in life as she did, or done so with such a radiant and sunny attitude. From the time she was five years old, when her mother was institutionalized and she was left with her aging grandfather, a rough old cob of a ranger at the newly opened Yellowstone National Park, until she died prematurely from pneumonia and other systems failures as a result of poliomyelitis, she was a happy person who always strived to make the most tasty lemonade from the sour citrus life had handed her.

A Vaudeville performer, actress, radio personality, artist, wife, mother of three, writer and poet, and work-at-home media critic (long before anyone ever heard of "telecommuting" and at a time when most married women—even the able-bodied—didn't work "outside" the home), Rainie made the most of every minute life gave her. She never forgot to practice the show business credo: "Always leave them smiling." I'm smiling still.

It's my privilege nearly 50 years after her death to present both her life and works. Her life was remarkable; her works—especially her poetry—are whimsical, philosophical, full of the joy, irony, and pathos of life, of careful observations of human strengths and weaknesses, the beauty of nature, and the contrariness of the human condition.

This book begins with a description of Rainie's life experience. It is not a full-scale biography, but a recollection and reconstruction based on available family and public information and the memories of her two surviving children. Inevita-

5

bly, much is missing, especially so since her husband, parents, and friends are almost all long gone.

Following the inspiring story of how she faced life's adversities are examples of the poetry she wrote in the 1950s and early 1960s and hoped to have published. In several cases, she wrote selections of poems around a theme that were intended to stand together; these are presented as separate "chapters."

Sadly, Rainie didn't live to see her children graduate from college, serve their country in the armed forces, embark on successful careers, marry and have children, and face all the struggles of life. Sadly, she also didn't live to see her poetry published. I am honored and privileged to remedy at least the latter omission with this volume.

Christopher M. Clarke
Huntingtown, Maryland
January 2011

Table of Contents

SMOKE AND MIRRORS:

Echoes From an Iron Lung

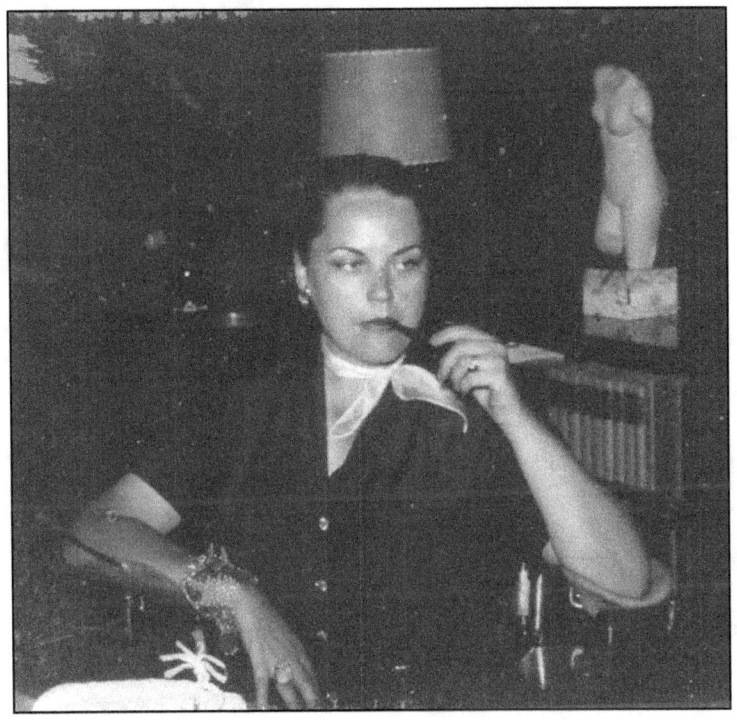

Previous page: Rainie Clarke at Warm Springs Foundation, 1956, in a pensive mood. Note that she is smoking a pipe, a reflection of her often independent-minded and iconoclastic attitude. In the early years after she returned home from Warm Springs, she sometimes smoked a corncob pipe rather than her usual (*Kool* brand) cigarettes.

A Tough First Act

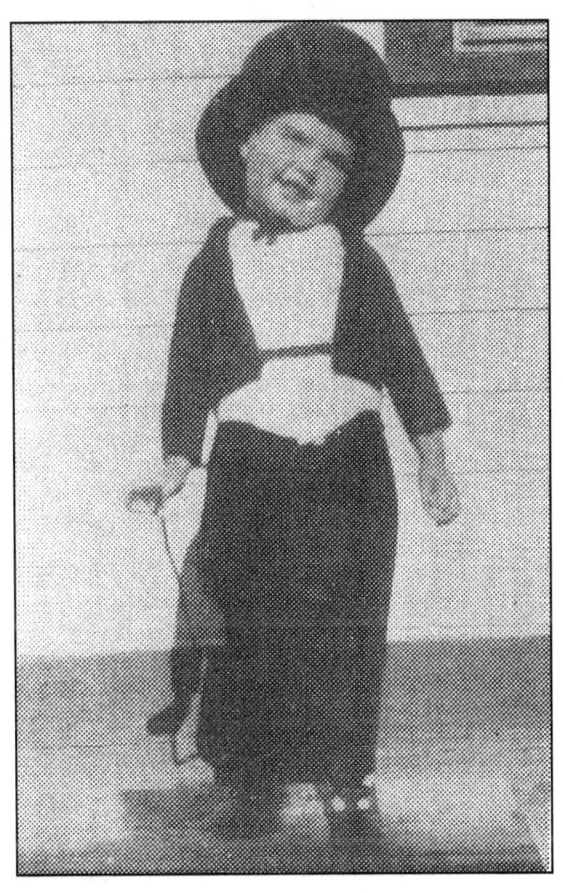

Previous page: A photo of Rainie at about age four in the cut-down tuxedo she sometimes wore in her parents' Vaudeville act.

I have no doubt that, given my mother's facility with words, the best way to introduce her story is to let her tell it herself:

I was born in Fort Worth, Texas; whelped of a theatrical family who were "at liberty" at the time (if one can be considered to be at liberty while in labor).[1] None of my ancestors escaped from debtors prison to flee on the Mayflower. They were all too busy stealing horses in Scotland, whence they were exiled to Ireland, being too much of a handful even for the hardy Celts.

Until I was four years old I trouped the southwestern vaudeville circuit with my folks, frequently making appearances at children's matinees. The uncertainty of life on the boards and another period of liberty led my mother to take me to live with my maternal grandfather.

This, of course, is only the bare bones of a much more interesting story. Rainie was born Lorraine Reynolds on November 28, 1920 to Frederick Alford Reynolds (1890-1972) and Grace Kathlyn ("Kitty") McFarland (1896-1929). Fred's ancestry can be traced with some certainty back to the time of the Crusades, a rather surprising fact given his unprepossessing nature, high-school education, hard-scrabble life and self-employment in a variety of ventures, and his descent from at least three generations of farmers.

Kitty McFarland's ancestors, on the other hand, disappear into the mist and myth of the Old Country. Her paternal grandparents were Irish immigrants from County Armagh and County Mayo who, like so many others, sought relief from the grinding poverty and strife by moving to the United States in the mid-19th century.

Both her grandfather and father, Harry McFarland (1869-1931), gravitated to the Army. Grandfather Peter (1818-1883) was a career soldier who served in some of the most God-forsaken out-

---

[1]. This section of autobiographical material is taken from an assignment Rainie Clarke fulfilled for a course in writing offered by *The Magazine Institute, Inc.* Unfortunately it is not dated but likely was written in 1956 or 1957. I have taken the liberty of occasionally rearranging the order of her narrative to better present her story.

posts of the Old West while dragging along a family of six boys and a girl. Harry spent most of his career as a mule packer, scout, and possibly a soldier in the Philippine Insurrection of 1899-1910. He ended his career, as we shall see, as a crew chief and head ranger at the newly established Yellowstone National Park in Wyoming.

Rainie's parents

Fred and Kitty eked out a living as Vaudeville performers.[2] Fred later related that when he was attending high school in Walla Walla, he traveled to and from school by means of a trolley that passed very near his house, but that because of the trolley schedule he was unable to stay after school and participate in any athletic or extra-curricular activities. Presumably wanting to escape the drudgery of farming and the small-town life he had grown up in, wanting to do something to "put myself forward," he decided to write a dramatic play. He and another "big country boy" who went to high school with Fred decided to collaborate on the production, which he planned to build around a plot involving "Prune" (a farmer's daughter), a villain, and a detective disguised as a farm hand.

Fred spent hours in a farm shed working on the details—plot, script, scenery, etc.—and decided that the only way he would be able to get an audience was to convince a school to sponsor the play. In order to do that, he offered to perform as a fund-raiser to purchase a piano for a local rural school. Having obtained the principal's permission, he visited the local Catholic school, which had a stock of ready-made scenery, and arranged to borrow some of it. Fred explained that he had utilized a little trickery to get permission for the play, leading the principal to believe that he had purchased the script and directions from a big firm that specialized in selling sheet music and ready-made plays for traveling troupes and local theater groups. Finally the big day arrived, and after numerous rehearsals, the play went on.

During the middle of the play, somehow the principal discovered that Fred had actually written the entire production. Rather than bring a halt to the show and chastise Fred, however, the princi-

---

[2] The following account is taken from a tape-recorded discussion between Fred and Rainie in 1958. I am grateful to Peter Craig for converting the original reel-to-reel tapes to digital media and providing me with a copy.

pal could see that the audience was thoroughly enjoying the performance, so at the intermission he announced that student Fred was
the author. It was so successful—both as entertainment and as a
fund-raiser—that the principal asked Fred and Co. to do a repeat
performance the next night. Thus began Fred A. Reynolds' career
in show business.

Leaving home?

After high school, probably about 1908, Fred decided to
take his act on the road and seek fame and fortune. He had saved up
a small amount of money, put together some "gags" from some of
the big Vaudeville shows, and with his friend, set off to "put himself
forward." Trying to break into the Western entertainment circuit of
traveling acts that moved from small town to small town in this age
before movies, Fred spent much of his money to purchase flamboy-
ant costumes in the style of entertainers of the time. He and his
partner decked themselves out in twin outfits of burnt-orange satin
suits with lavender lapels and long coats.

Somehow, through exuding self-confidence and a little
creative story-telling, Fred convinced an agent to give him a chance.
By happenstance, the agent needed an additional act for a Vaudeville show in Everett, Washington. Fred and his partner hopped on
the train and showed up at the little theater, prepared to add their act
to the show. The afternoon of their first performance, they received
their cue and stepped on stage to do a little dance number in front of
about 30 paying matinee customers. But just as they began, the coal
delivery man arrived and began to shovel coal for the furnace down
the metal chute right next to the stage, making such a racket that he
threw them off their timing and drowned out their act. Fred realized
that they "hadn't made the grade," and sure enough, they were fired.

In those days, performers received no pay for their first
show. Only if they passed muster and were retained did they get a
pay check. So Fred and Co., having spent all their money to get to
Everett dressed in style, were destined to be stranded and broke.
The theater manager, however, took pity on the young would-be
Vaudevillians and bought each of them a ticket back to Seattle. In
Seattle, they wired home for money for a ticket back to Walla
Walla. By the time they had spent their last 15 cents for dinner,
they arrived home with a nickel in their pocket, a bit wiser in the

ways of the world and with a much better appreciation for the difficulties of "putting yourself forward" in show business.

Working the small time circuit

Undiscouraged, Fred went to work in a hotel in Walla Walla. He took a job as an "illustrated singer," showing slides as he sang along. While hanging around a pool hall, a shoe-shiner introduced Fred to a fellow named "Mal," who would become his traveling and show business partner for the next few years.[3] Mal had been working in Seattle as a singer and was doing a gig in Walla Walla. The two decided to join their acts together and try to break into the "circuit," a round of small-town appearances scheduled and arranged by a manager. All they had to offer was a few songs by Mal and a few comedy routines Fred could perform.

They booked an appearance in a small town on the edge of Idaho to be paid with a percentage of the revenue. They seem to have done alright, because the manager wanted to engage them for another week on the condition that they present a new show for the extension. They worked with a piano player—almost every small town had a piano player who played along with the newest entertainment invention, the silent movie—and the stage manager to develop a bigger repertoire.

The stage manager taught them some new jokes and how to pantomime playing dice and poker, and they added new opening and closing song-and-dance routines. One of their pantomimes was copied from a well-known Vaudevillian, Bert Williams—stealing others' acts and jokes was a routine part of the business—about learning how to be a waiter serving wine.

The pair began a grueling round of the small towns of a still poor and frontier west: Nez Perce, Twin Falls, Boise, and numerous whistle stops between and beyond. They dropped the gaudy costumes and began to perform stock-character comedy sketches; in Fred's words, Mal played the "smart nigger" in a satin suit and Fred played the "bum nigger" whose poor command of English and *faux*

[3.] Unfortunately I have been unable to find any additional information—including a full name—about "Mal," but he and Fred remained friends for many years even after leaving show business.

pas and prat falls were a staple of Vaudeville.[4]

Not all went smoothly on the road to fame and fortune. Fred and Mal played towns such as Shoshone, Idaho—a "rough town" full of sheep-herders—Salt Lake City, and Evanston, Wyoming. Well, not Evanston. On the train headed in that direction, the two met a show operator who promised them a job when they got there, but when they arrived, there was no job available. They were broke, without even the money to get out of town and try to find another gig down the railroad.

Finally, in desperation, Mal, a member of the Moose Lodge fraternity, gave the secret Moose disaster signal. An old rancher recognized his Lodge "brother" and gave the pair a dollar to pay the hotel bill they had already incurred and told them to go get their suitcases, which the hotel had been holding as surety against the bill. A couple of railroad men treated them to a meal and one of the conductors offered to put their suitcases on the train headed east. He told Fred and Mal that if the conductor got the assignment to the east-bound train, he'd make sure they got on board. Something went wrong and their luggage headed down the tracks without them. Fred and Mal wound up hitching a ride on a freight train to Green River, Wyoming after learning from some hoboes how to avoid getting caught (and beat up) by the railroad guards and where the best place was to jump the train (where it had to slow down on an incline).

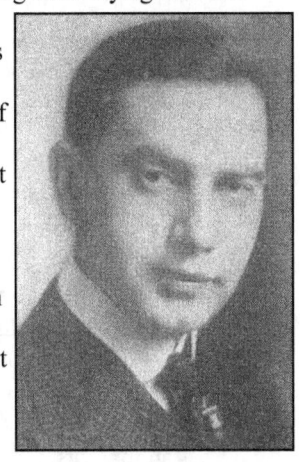

A young Fred Reynolds

Fred's narrative gave only some examples of the rough life on the road, but also repeatedly showed the kindness and generosity of strangers. In one incident, he and his partner were stranded in a desolate area, hoping to catch a ride on a passing train. Nothing was in view but a single house, apparently belonging to the railroad em-

---

[4] This was the language Fred used. One has to remember that even well after this period, such famous performers as Al Jolson made their careers by performing "black face" comedy.

ployee responsible for manning the water tower and guarding against train-jumpers. The owners treated him kindly and gave him something to eat.

Fred finds a wife

After beating around on the informal Western Vaudeville circuit with modest success, Fred decided to return to Walla Walla, probably around 1915 or 1916. As he told Rainie in a letter dated February 17, 1958:

> In my early days I went back home to visit Walla Walla to visit what people were left that raised and schooled me. A member of the family had opened a pool hall and cigar store and asked me to stay and help him run it with a future partnership in the future. So I stayed put that winter and met your mother [ed. Kitty McFarland] at some nice party of young people. She was the musician of the bunch and played the piano while the rest horsed around.
>
> She was living with her grand parents at the time and didn't know her father or mother. Her mother was dead at that time and I didn't know any of her background and right now I'm having trouble dredging up the name of her grandparents. I only saw them a couple of times. They were lovely people. He was a veterinarian for the 7th or 14th Cavalry stationed at Fort Walla Walla. [Note: The family was John and Mary Tempany.] Your mother had a brother, George. I believed [sic.] he was also raised by the grandparents.
>
> Well as the winter wore on, Kitty and I fell in love and became engaged. The understanding was that I was to go back to the Southwest where I could make connections in show business and send for her at the oportune [sic. opportune] moment and get married. So we were married in Muskogee in 1918. Dunn and Brandon, a vaudeville team, stood for us with the Justice of the Peace. Incidentally, we formed a foursome.

18

Your mother [Kitty] to my mind was a great musician, one of the few naturals.[5] She played with such effortless ease in a lilting sort of way. She was born with that talent. She had studied music and could play the classics when called to do so. But she didn't care too much for them. She reveled in current music of our time. She was great on the piano—her first love. Next she tried the Sax and in a few weeks became so proficient she could sit in any orchestra. I've seen her horsing around with music for her own amusement—sit down to the piano with her sax strapped around her neck and grasped in her right hand, beat the piano with her left, and finger the sax with her right, playing a different tune with each instrument simultaneously. I can recall one of the tunes was "Dixie" but I can't recall the other.

Any time an actor wandered onto the show and turned up for rehearsal without music, having lost it somewhere along the line, she would sit down to the piano and say simply, 'Hum it!'

In fifteen minutes she would have his numbers down and playing like mad, and a surprised and pleased actor. One day she remarked she would like to have a piano accordion. So I bought her a beautiful one for $450.00 [note: a huge amount of money at the time] and in a short time she mastered it to the point of doing specialties.

In Jan 1925 I took over management of [the] Tabloid musical, "Honeymoon Misses," on the Gus Suntime for Harvey Dorr home office, Kokomo, Ind. I was road manager and also participated in the general activities. Your mother did her accordion specialty. She also sang with it. She inclined toward Blues numbers. She had a low, pleasing voice, not much volume but she held her own and always

---

5. The following paragraphs are from a letter from Fred to Rainie dated June 29, 1958.

got honorable mentions in the write-ups. Well at that time "Sally" was new and a big number. All vaudeville and tab(loid) shows were using it.[6]

So we made a big spec out of it, Sally sitting on the park bench. At the finish, the cop comes and escorts her to jail. Your mother played the accordion for the number and I was the mean old Cop. Now the reason for your seeing this—Every week I sent an ad in advance to the next stand: "Wanted for week, high school girl [to] act as maid. Call at Bijou between hours 9 and 11 Monday morning." Well, needless to say, there were always 10 to 15 girls on hand. We would pick the most likely one to squire you [Lorraine, age 3-4] for the week and keep you out of our hair during rehearsals and performances. And I will add, we had some lovely girls who fell in love with you and wanted to travel with us, which was of course impossible.

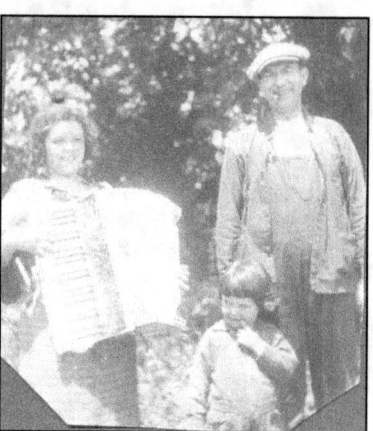

I would give them a ticket or pass for the Sat. matinee and have them bring you along. The first performance you attended, you dis-tracted the actor and audience by shouting at my first appearance, "That's my Daddy!" We cautioned the maids and you thereaf-ter to simmer down which you did. Incidentally, you cost us our job on that show (a

Kitty, Lorraine, and Fred Reynolds about 1924.

tent show), the Edith Ambler Show. The story goes like this. The Reynolds had closed with some show, name for-gotten, and were hanging around Chicago. An agent

---

[6.] A "tabloid" show was an abbreviated version of a full-sized show put on in big cities like New York.

booked us out on this dramatic tent show early in the spring [in] some town in Illinois. We played a string of small hamlets.

Your mother was musical director and I Gen(eral) Bus (iness)—and specialties between acts. This show put on a Sat matinee for children. Red Ridinghood was the Spec (ialty). Mr. Ambler ask[ed] me if he could advertise and use you as a walk-on specialty between acts. It being the afternoons, we agreed—you were 4 years old and we had cut down one of my old evening dress suits to fit you. High plug hat and all.

The big moment came. Your mother played you on and I gave you a shove from the wings, and out you went, trooper that you were. [You] did a few wobbly steps half out of time then turned your prat to the audience and gave a slow elaborate bow.

The audience applauded and howled. You stopped the show. This gave the manager an idea—every Sat nite he gave a penny snatching after show following the main performance. He sold extra tickets and candy—the prize box kind. We actors put on our jackets and passed the candy out, 10% our cut. Well he got the idea he wanted to advertise you for the late show, which closed about mid-night. Well at your age we saw that you got to bed every night no later than 9 o'clock. We cared more for your health than what the manager wanted. We explained about your tender age and the late hours. The manager said Okay, and in a few days we received our two weeks notice.

We didn't give a hang as we felt we had right on our side.

So this was the crazy, exciting, but hardly stable or conventional life of Rainie's first four or five years. Unfortunately, the idyll was about to come to a crashing end. In Rainie's words, "The uncertainty of life on the boards and another period of liberty led my mother to take me to live with my maternal grandfather," in 1925.

While visiting Harry McFarland, then retired from service with the Army and serving as a ranger and crew chief at Yellowstone National Park, and preparing to leave her child there, Kitty suffered a mental breakdown. Psychiatry in those days remained primitive, but it became increasingly clear that Kitty was seriously ill and required hospitalization. In the later words of Rainie, "Grandpa consulted many doctors. Finally, with sorrow, he had my mother, a young victim of schizophrenia, committed to the Montana State Hospital. There four years later, with-out regaining her sanity, she died."[7]

From pillar to post

Rainie explained what happened next:

Since a four year old female can create problems for a footloose, rough-hewn old westerner, I was boarded out. When this proved unsuccessful Grandfather allowed friends, a Mr. and Mrs. Whittaker, to take me to Miami, Florida, for the winter. Their ultimate aim, I believe, was to adopt me, but their plans were to be frustrated. Show business was on the rocks and my own father had gravitated to the Everglades where his dad owned a shack on some homestead property. When Father heard that I was in Miami with "strangers", he borrowed a car, drove to Miami and demanded immediate possession of his daughter. The Whittakers had no alternative but to comply.

Apparently Fred coaxed his daughter with promises of a magical life in a mystical Paradise called Canal Point. Paradise turned out to be rather different than she expected, however.

I remember the drive up the Tamiami Trail: miles of scrubby wilderness, punctuated occasionally by the bril-

---

[7] It's not clear what Fred was thinking in deciding to leave little Lorraine with her Grandfather. Harry's wife had divorced him years earlier and unable to care for his own children, he had sent them to be raised by their maternal grandparents, the Tempanys, in Walla Walla, Washington. It should have been clear that this arrangement could never have worked out.

22

liant plumage of startled birds. Father's campaign strategy was superb. He simply reckoned without the lively imagination of a five year old. He promised school, playmates and frequent visits from beloved 'Daddy'. He told of lush green fields and vivid flowers, a sparkling lake and fishing every day!—a veritable Nirvana.

The name of Nirvana was Canal Point. The town (and I say it with a smile, Mister) consisted of four weather-beaten shacks and one hash house separated from two weather-beaten shacks, a boarding house and a newspaper office by canal locks and an iron bridge. It stood at the point where the Florida canal system empties into Lake Okeechobee. There were no children, no lush green fields except for the bean crops, and no sidewalks. The huddled little community looked like a fat sow wallowing in a sea of mud.

Father had the restaurant concession in the hash house, which also doubled as bar room and billiard parlor. I was not allowed to visit it.

Again I was boarded out; this time in the boarding house across the locks. This establishment was owned and operated by a Mrs. Barrett. She catered to itinerant crop pickers, traveling salesmen and an occasional fishing party from Palm Beach. Mrs. Barrett was a generous, warmhearted woman who knew very little about children. She must have felt sorry for me, for she agreed to board me for the cost of my milk and very little money, in exchange for which I was to make myself as useful as possible. I soon learned to sweep, to make beds and to set the table. My most memorable chore, however, dealt with cleaning up a sleeping porch on the second floor. This was the room where Mrs. Barrett's invalid, insane and incontinent sister slept.

My days were not entirely devoted to chores. I made mud pies (the supply always outlasting the demand), pedaled my tricycle and, on Sunday, enjoyed the luxury of a free funny paper from the newspaper office next door. When Mrs. Barrett's sister did not occupy the shadowy fumed oak dining room, counting her fingers and cackling like a brooder hen, I stole into it and spent hours playing the gramophone. I danced for a faintly remembered audience, and sang the lyrics of the only record in the house -- "The Mademoiselle From Armentieres".

It was on just such an afternoon that a charming little woman from Palm Beach wandered into the dining room and formed an appreciative gallery of one. Her name was Mrs. Woodruff and she had come out with a fishing party. She had noticed me before, but always under the misconception that I was a boy. When the mistake had been corrected, she first consulted with Mrs. Barrett, and then with my father; whereupon she invited me to spend two weeks with her in Palm Beach. In my limited experience this was the first time being a girl had paid off.

Inevitably, the two weeks spread to the summer and the summer melted into fall. Grandfather [Ed.: Harry McFarland] made a hasty trip to Florida to investigate the Woodruffs. It was on his insistence that Father finally agreed to let the Woodruffs adopt me. So in a sense I moved from the squalor of the Everglades to the opulence of Palm Beach on the strength of my sex and the lyrics of a ribald song.

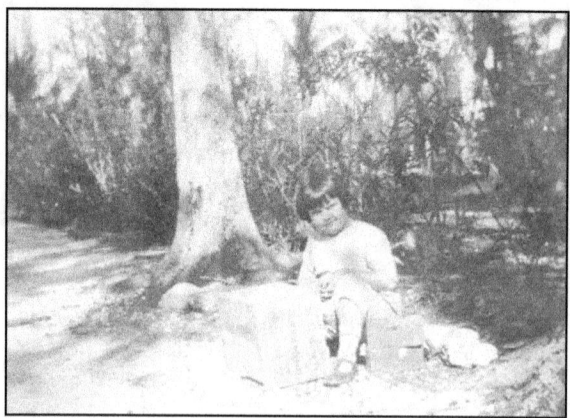

Blissful Interlude

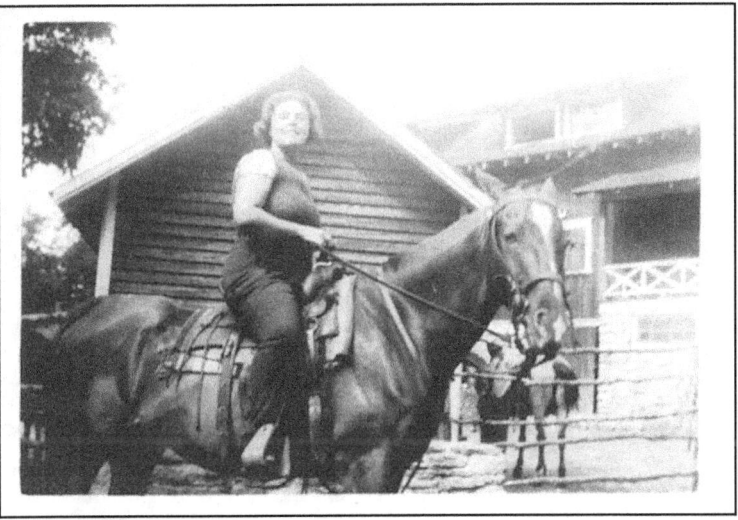

Previous page: Rainie at about age 17, riding her favorite horse, "Pure Gold," at Claw's Dude Ranch in Florida, August 1937.

Rainie (then known as Lorraine) was to thrive in the world of Palm Beach for more than the next decade under the loving care of her ageing and childless adoptive parents, Harry Clarence Woodruff (1869-1942) and his wife Daisy (1874-1940). Unfortunately, however, Rainie left little concrete information about life with the Woodruffs other than a number of photos, and genealogical research has been unsuccessful in turning up much about the family.

Harry (possibly born Henry) was the son of William I. Woodruff, born about 1846 in Kentucky, and Ellen, whose maiden name I have not been able to uncover, who was born about 1849 in Illinois. They were of modest circumstances, living in Cook County and Christian County, Illinois. William was a laborer who worked his way up to office clerk, and Ellen worked as a milliner. William died sometime before 1920, but I have found no record of Ellen's passing.

Harry grew up in Illinois, but at some point apparently moved to New York City where he began a career as a businessman. He apparently made a considerable fortune in business, though I have been unable to discover what kind of business he was engaged in. In 1910 he was a manager of a "supply house," and had bought a house in Queens on mortgage. At the age of 40, he was well enough off to have a servant, a 19-year-old Virginia girl who lived with the family.

It is likely that Harry's business involved at least some import and export, as in 1920 he and his wife, Daisy, traveled to Argentina, Brazil, and Chile for "commercial and business" purposes aboard the *S.S. Vauban*, according to their passport application. They apparently had never traveled abroad before because this was their first passport application. They returned to New York on the *Essequibo* on April 19, 1921.

By 1930, at age 60, Harry had made his fortune and retired, moving to Palm Beach, Florida, where the couple apparently lived quite well. Their household included not only Harry, Daisy, and the recently adopted Lorraine, but a male servant; Celeste Murray, 63, a "sister-in-law"; Daisy I. Morgan, 43, a niece; Powers P. Murray, 26, a nephew who worked as a bank clerk; and Margaret Bowles, 14, a great niece.

Harry was married to Daisy Estelle, whose maiden name I was unable to discover. She was born in Virginia in 1874, apparently to a well-off family. Her father seems to have emigrated from England, but her mother was a native Virginian. They may have been associated with the Richmond Hotel, as a number of pieces of fine silverware from that establishment were passed down to Rainie in the Woodruff's estate.[1] It is not clear how Harry and Daisy met, but they were married in 1894, when he was about 26 and she was about 20.

I have been unable to uncover much information about Harry and Daisy's retired life in Florida, but they seem to have been part of the expanding East Coast elite that had taken up residence in the developing exclusive environs of South Florida. The family owned a large yacht which they used for boating and fishing and were active in the swanky and exclusive Sailfish Club of Florida, which had been organized in February 1914. Harry may have been an early member of the Club; in 1931 he was elected chairman of the House Committee (apparently the chief executive office) and a member of the Board of Directors. Among the few possessions Lorraine inherited from the Woodruffs were several pieces of silver, including at least one tray from the Sailfish Club, an award for a fishing competition.

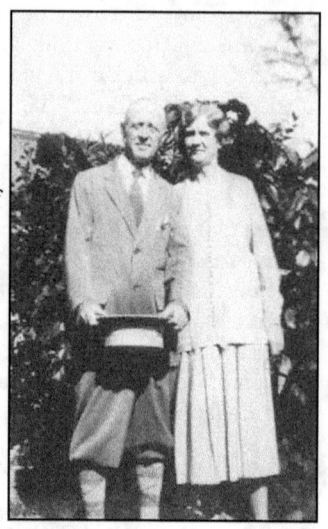

Harry and Daisy Woodruff
About 1926

A youth of relative privilege

The Woodruffs provided numerous opportunities for Lorraine, including vacations at a Dude Ranch and a home within walking distance of the beach. Little information remains about

---

[1.] The provenance of this silverware—including pitchers and other tableware for fine dining—is uncertain. There was also a "Richmond Hotel" in Palm Beach during the period when the Woodruffs lived there, and they may have acquired the pieces there.

these activities other than a collection of photos Rainie kept over the years. (See following pages.) As she grew older, Lorraine became both an excellent student and an outstanding swimmer. Despite her tendency to possess a "full figure," she swam several miles each morning with the local lifeguards in the sometimes rough Atlantic Ocean waters. She appears to have been a vivacious, outgoing, and relatively popular girl through high school.

Storm clouds were brewing over her tropical paradise, however. According to Rainie, writing more than two decades later, the stock market crash of 1929 and the ensuing Great Depression virtually wiped out the Woodruff's wealth. In her words:

> Memories of that earlier Palm Beach are still vivid, as are the now familiar terms of "Boom" and "Crash" which seasoned all grown-up conversations. I did not understand the words at the time. I only knew that our cabin cruiser had sunk in a hurricane and, as Mrs. Woodruff put it, our ship was no longer coming in.

Despite their reduced financial circumstances, the Woodruffs apparently were still well enough off to afford Lorraine a number of opportunities. In the summer of 1935, for example, she attended Camp Carlysle, apparently in Florida, where she seems to have served as a camp counselor. Existing photos suggest she may have taught swimming and that she engaged in horseback riding and theatrical productions. In the summer of 1937, she attended Claw's Dude Ranch where she continued with horseback riding and other activities.

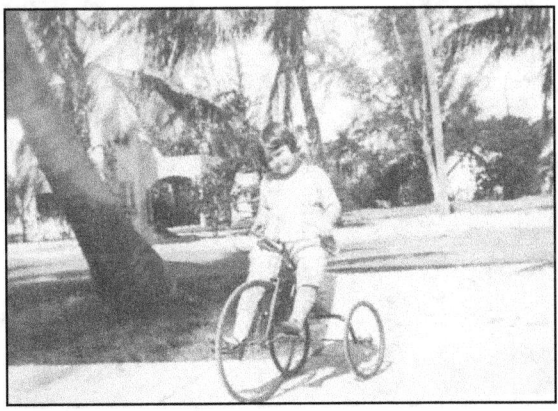

Lorraine Woodruff as a teenager, camp counselor, and high school graduate during the 1930s.

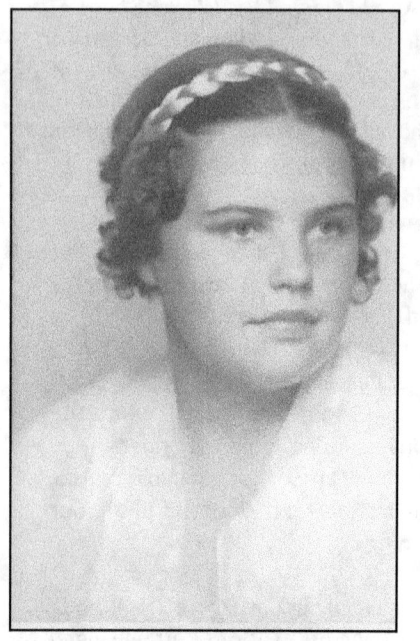

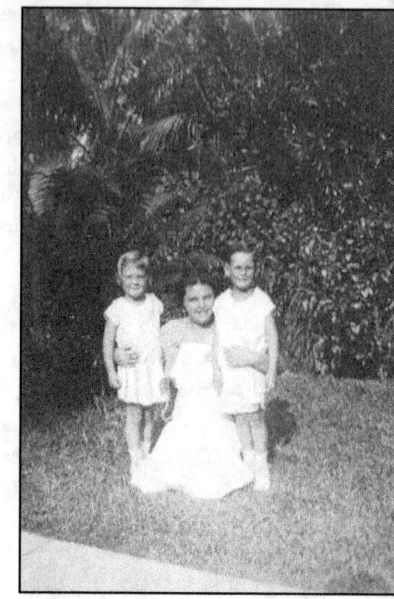

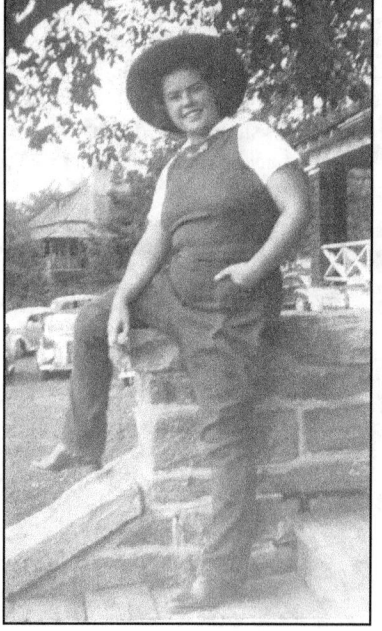

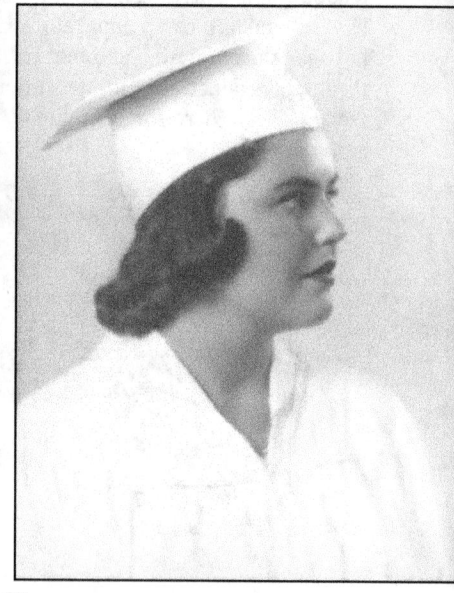

Off to the Big City

Lorraine graduated from Palm Beach High School in 1938 and in the fall moved to New York to attend the two-year American Academy of Dramatic Arts. Her own autobiographical sketch explains the circumstances:

> My first ambitious sights were trained on an operatic career, and I rent the air in our neighborhood with vocal scales for years before I realized that my singing coach ... had successfully ruined the promising voice of a beginner. One is not born of Scotch-Irish ancestry for nothing. I shed the disappointment like dead skin and settled for the next best goal--the theater.

> The financial misfortunes of the Woodruffs had cast a pall over the brilliant educational possibilities which had been forecast for me. Once again Grandfather [Harry McFarland] came to my rescue, albeit posthumously, [he died in 1931] when his bequest paid my tuition to The American Academy of Dramatic Arts in Carnegie Hall.

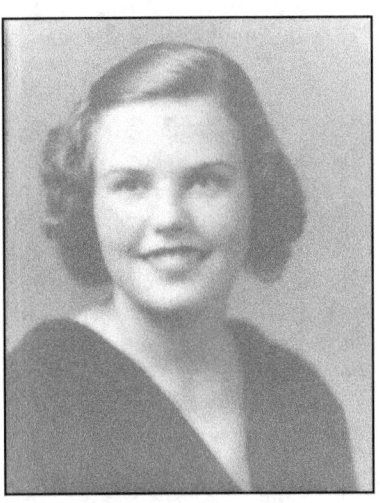

Rainie about 1937.

> I spent two winters at the Academy in New York, living the Gay Life and feeling very Bohemian.

Lorraine apparently took full advantage of her time in New York both to study drama and to enjoy herself. Living with roommate Helen Slidell, the two spent a good deal of time—often with male companions—seeing the sights. Again, however, she left little

31

testimony of her activities, but a considerable photographic record. (See pages 35-36.) By this time, she was becoming known as "Rainie," a nickname she apparently took up at least partly as a stage name.[2]

Turning points

The summer of 1939, half-way through her matriculation at the dramatic arts academy, proved to be a crucial one for Rainie. She returned to Palm Beach where she looked for opportunities to practice her new craft of drama. During that summer, as she later told the story, "I was introduced to John Clarke, an announcer at our local radio station." In a later publicity release, Rainie explained that they met "over a hot microphone, [and] she and Johnny Clarke teamed for an 'informal chatter show' on WJNO," where Clarke was working.[3] According to Rainie, "His first words were, 'How do you do? Will you marry me?'"

Rainie and John apparently spent much of the summer together, with her doing several daily spot announcements on WJNO[4] for various women's shops; co-hosting a half-hour daily variety show with John which included chit-chat, discussions of styles, recipes, cooking hints, movie reviews, society news, current events, human interest stories, interviews, and music. Rainie also wrote and was featured in a 15-minute weekly program of household hints and home decoration tips. Simultaneously, she was assistant director of the dramatic department of the Society of Four Arts in Palm Beach.

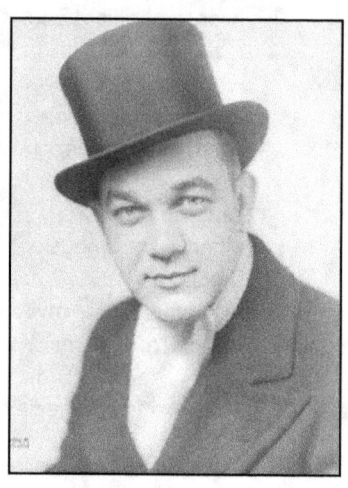

Johnny Clarke, about 1939.

---

[2] She may also have used "Rainie" to avoid being confused with Laraine Day, a famous movie star who was also born in the fall of 1920.

[3] The term "hot microphone" meant one that was broadcasting live, but the double-entendre was clearly intended.

[4] WJNO, a CBS affiliate, was the only major radio station between Orlando and Miami, drawing 94% of the listening audience, according to polling at the time.

Rainie still had a year to finish at the Academy in New York, and she returned there in the fall. Upon graduation, she returned to Palm Beach where, in 1940, she wrote all newspaper and radio copy for a chain of women's shops, narrated all their style shows, and wrote and narrated daily 15-minute programs on style and society for WJNO. She also became the managing director of the Theater Workshop and Norton Galleries.

John, meanwhile, had accepted a position as a staff announcer and producer at WRBL in Columbus, Georgia. While apart, tragedy was to strike the Woodruff household in 1940. At the age of 66, Rainie's adoptive mother, Daisy, died suddenly and unexpectedly on June 28. Rainie described the circumstances in a heart-broken letter to her fiancé on July 2:

> Dearest, Up until now I haven't been able to write, but now I think perhaps I can...Poor darling [Harry Woodruff], he's so crushed, it's just heart breaking to watch him. He and mother had been married 45 years. 46 this August...
>
> Last Thursday morning I left the house about 12:30—mother was feeling better than usual and quite cheerful, tho' she thought it to [sic.] hot to go out—so I went to the hospital to see Daisy [a niece] - then to visit some friends. I returned about 2:45 and found mother on the living room couch complaining of a terrible headache and pain through her eye.
>
> I got some cracked ice to see if it would relieve the pain. She then became terribly nauseated and I took her upstairs. I made her lie down and noticed she was becoming weaker. I helped her into the bathroom 3 or 4 times—the last time she was so weak that I had to pick her up and support her. At the time I noticed something but was so upset that I paid no attention to it. She seemed to limp on her left leg.
>
> I undressed her, put on her nightgown, then got the electric fan. She seemed to be resting much more easily and I stayed right beside her asking her every so often how she felt. She would say, "a little better" and then would ask for some water. I begged her to let me call a doctor, but she refused. (She never has had faith in them and didn't seem to feel that she needed one.)

About quarter after twelve, Dad went upstairs to bed—felt mother's pulse. It was beating regularly and she was breathing easily. So he went to sleep feeling sure that she would be all right in the morning. I must have had a premonition of it for I never closed my eyes that entire night. I looked in the room several times during the night and mother was apparently all right. I came downstairs about 3:30 and sat until five when I decided to go for a swim.

I returned from the beach about 7:30 and was just at the corner when I saw my cousin coming for me. Of course I realized immediately what had happened. Dad woke up a [t] five after seven and called to mother saying "Doll, we're late for the war news." There was no answer—and then he discovered what had happened. She had been dead for several hours, as she was very cold and rigor mortis had set in. There was no struggle as she was in the same position as when Dad went to bed. I would have heard her had she made any noise. She passed on in her sleep. The Doctor said had we called him he could have done nothing. I am so thankful she suffered none. She was the only person in her family who passed on without a long serious illness.

Apparently Daisy's death caught Rainie at a vulnerable time. In mid-June, shortly before her mother died, Rainie had written John a melancholy letter questioning whether he was still interested in her, complaining of the distance and lack of contact, and bemoaning his infrequent letter-writing. They appear to have moved beyond this rough patch, aided in part by John's sympathetic response to Daisy's death, and in 1941, Rainie moved to Columbus, Georgia where the two were married on October 18, 1941.[4]

[4.] Harry Woodruff died in 1942, but I have found little documentation among John and Rainie's effects to indicate their reaction. Given her attachment to Harry—whom she always called her father—it must have been difficult to lose him so soon after losing her mother, but being married and with her husband likely cushioned the blow. Having lost so much of their fortune during the Depression, Harry does not appear to have left much of an estate to his adopted daughter. There is no record of her having received any substantial amount of money, though she did inherit some personal belongings, including fine linens and silver pieces (trays, pitchers, etc.)

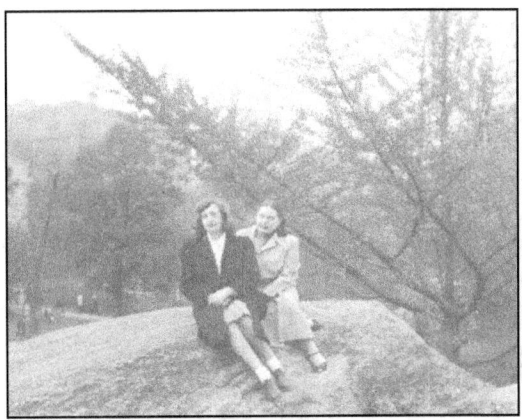

In Central Park with roommate,
Helen Slidell.

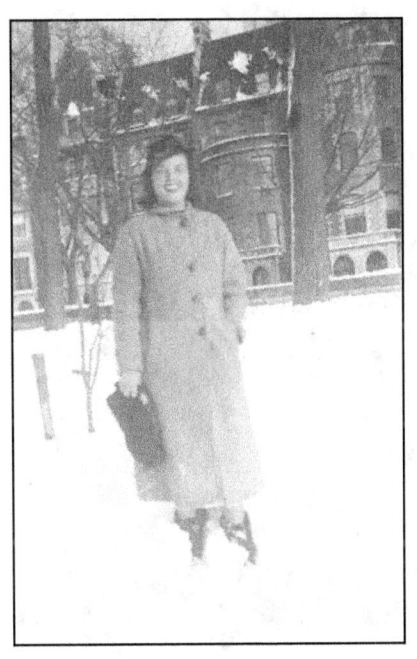

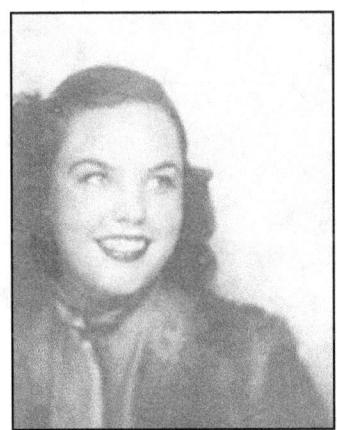

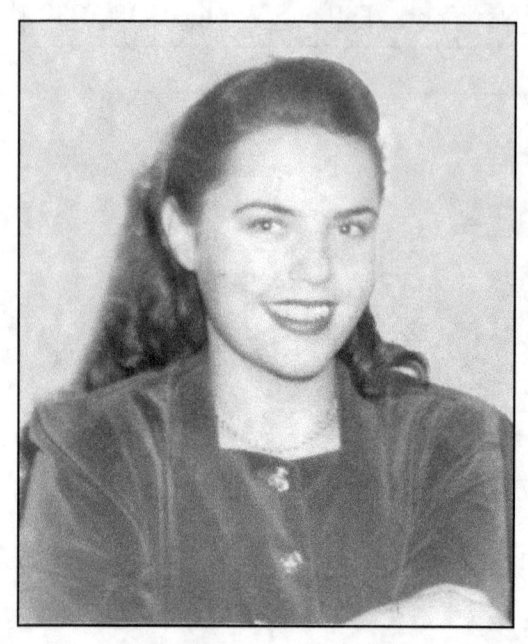

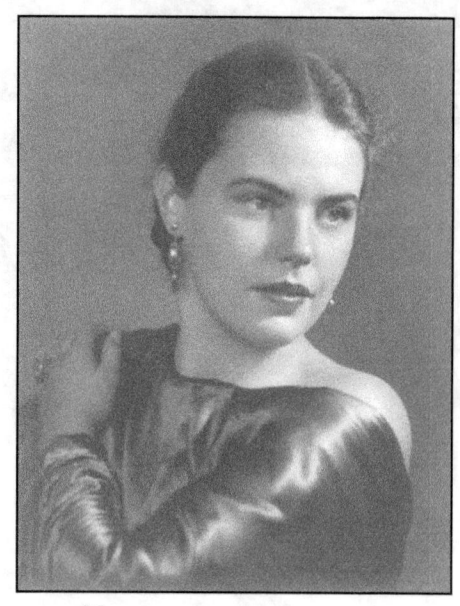

The Wartime Years

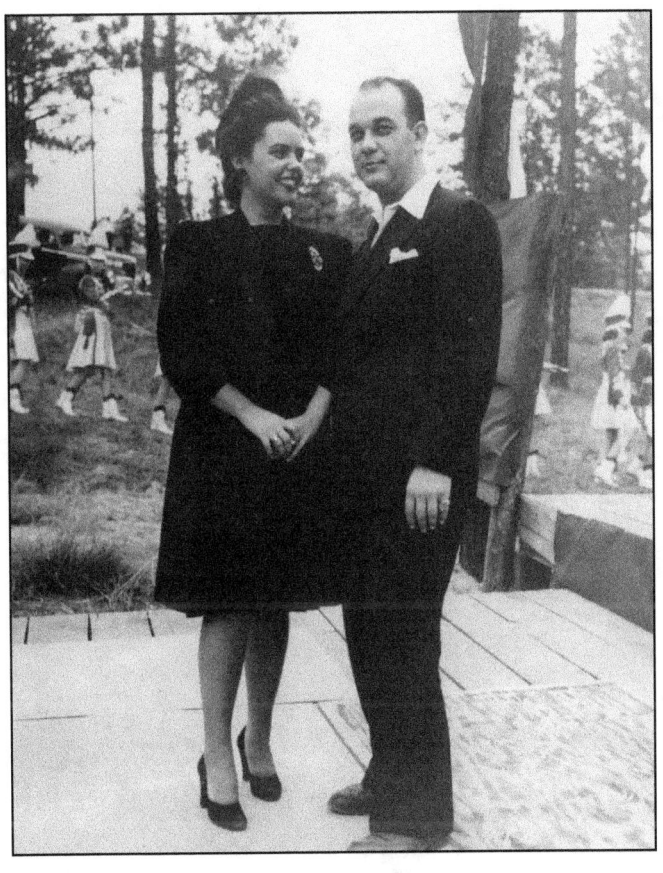

Previous page: John and Rainie Clarke shortly after their marriage
in 1941.

J ohn and Rainie's wedding, like so much of their life, turned out to be an adventure coupled with zany problems. Rainie later told the story:

> We applied for our license in Muskogee county, but we were married by an army chaplain in the post chapel [at Fort Benning] which was, of course, government property. At the time it did not seem complicated. However, I misplaced (permanently, as it turned out) our wedding certificate. A year later when John entered the service, I had a very embarrassing time trying to convince Uncle Sam that we had not been living in sin. The only official record of our wedding was with an army chaplain, hip deep in Italian mud.

John spent from 1939 to the spring of 1943 as production manager for WRBL, the key station for the Georgia Broadcasting System, located in Columbus, Georgia. For three years, he was loaned by the station to Fort Benning and was in charge of all theatrical and radio activities for the post. This included producing 17 weekly Vaudeville programs and 14 weekly radio broadcasts featuring all-soldier talents. John interviewed candidates, developed the shows, wrote the material, ran rehearsals, and narrated the shows. During this period he also wrote, produced, and narrated the first Army Hour from the Army-Navy YMCA in Columbus. This series was cited in September 1940 by Radio Digest as the most outstanding of its type, and John received commendations for his exemplary work from both the Joint Army-Navy Welfare Committee and the U.S. Army. He was cited by the U.S. Treasury Department for selling $110,000 in bonds in one 45 minute show.

Rainie was almost equally busy. In addition to serving as John's assistant director-producer for radio and theatrical entertainment at Fort Benning, she did daily spot radio announcements for several women's shops, co-hosted a quiz show on WRBL, and was producer-director, script supervisor, and narrator for a weekly half-hour radio show by the Little Theater of Columbus. The two also were featured for three years as "Mr. and Mrs. Santa Claus" on WRBL.

Perhaps as important as her professional contributions was her role as hostess-in-chief for John in his capacity as radio and entertainment personality and head of entertainment for Fort Benning. As she later remembered it, with her usual sense of humor:

> I spent the first year of our marriage learning that an army travels on its stomach and your victuals. If John and I wanted to be alone, we had to leave a case of beer on our kitchen table, the front door open, and retire to the officer's club at the post. At one time or another, we entertained everybody in the Second Armored Division except General Patton, and I think John picked up his bar tab once or twice.

In the late summer of 1942—the low point in the Allied war effort—John and Rainie took a brief vacation in New York. As John later described it: "While [in New York], I made up my mind that I was soon going into the Army [and] consequently turned down a job with OWI [Office of War Information] here. We went to Columbus [Ohio] for a football game and to visit my kid brother who lives on a farm in Central Ohio. Rainie and I both liked Columbus...so we decided to settle there while I was in the Army." The next year proved to be turbulent—and nearly fatal for John.

Off to war?

For some reason, John had difficulty being released by the Georgia draft board so he could enlist in Columbus, Ohio. While waiting for his release, he did some work for WCOL, but by around the end of 1942, his release had come through. In March 1943, he was sent to the "reception center" at Fort Benjamin Harrison in Indiana for induction. At the reception center, inductees were issued their basic kits (clothes, boots, etc.) and taught some fundamentals such as marching in formation and military courtesy, before receiving an onward assignment to another camp for basic training. Some, like John, were also selected for "other duties." In John's case, this was assisting the supply sergeant in issuing and keeping track of all linens and other bedding temporarily issued to inductees. Most inductees shipped out relatively quickly, but John was stuck at Ft. Harrison for roughly a month.

Eventually, John was assigned to Camp Blanding, Florida, where a brand new division, the 66th, was forming. In his words, "It was a rugged outfit. We got basic and Ranger training concurrently." It was such a "rugged outfit" because, without the personnel knowing it, the 66th was training for the D-Day invasion.

John applied to join the Special Services branch, which included entertainment programming. In what apparently was a highly unusual arrangement, he simultaneously participated *both* in the military training regimen *and* ran entertainment programs for the Camp. His wartime letters show he was holding down a brutal schedule. As he later remembered it, "During this time I was doing two half-hour broadcasts per week, which I had to write, cast, produce, and narrate. There were 12 Vaudeville shows weekly to cast, rehearse and mc [emcee, or Master of Ceremonies]. All of this activity along *with basic.* Long rugged hikes, sleepless nights, and overwork."

John's letters at the time show that he was also dealing with an extremely difficult commanding officer, a Captain whom no

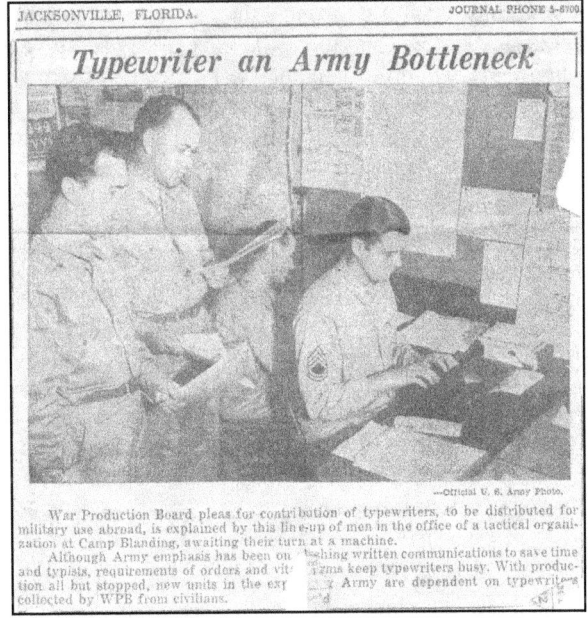

The only known photo of John Clarke (second from left) in U.S. Army uniform, 1943.

41

one apparently liked or respected, who worked his men like dogs, and who took all the credit for successes while blaming any shortcomings on his subordinates. A testimony to the excellent work John was doing, however, was his promotion directly from buck private to Technical Sergeant Fourth Class (T-4), the first such promotion in the 66th Division. He also received considerable personal attention from both the Colonel and Commanding General above him. Finally, the grueling pace in the Florida heat and humidity and the constant stress of dealing with his commanding officer overtook John.

> I started losing weight. Fell out on a hike and was sent to the hospital [apparently on or about July 18] where I had a complete breakdown and was very ill for several weeks. After spending four months in the hospital and losing 100 pounds, I was [honorably] discharged and returned to Columbus [Ohio].

John's letters from the hospital indicate that the doctors really didn't know what was wrong with him. He had chronic diarrhea, couldn't hold down any food, was excessively sensitive to light or noise, and couldn't sleep but was so tired he couldn't do anything. His letters show that he was embarrassed by his "weakness" and concerned that, if discharged, others would look down on him as a shirker or malingerer.

Of course, Rainie was hundreds of miles away and couldn't come to his aid. Moreover, the newly-weds were financially strapped, with John's meager Army pay not even covering basic expenses. As only John's letters seem to have been preserved, it is difficult to reconstruct Rainie's life and troubles during this trying time. She later wrote:

> While my husband was in service, I worked, first as a salesgirl in a department store, and later as a credit investigator for The Household Finance Corporation. I was one of the first women they had employed for "outside" work. During my tenure with them I was offered a job with the FBI which I tactfully refused. Now that I look back on it, I doubt if the FBI job would have been as dangerous as the one I was doing.

Although I have been unable to uncover specifics, Rainie was also undergoing problems, apparently including some friction with John's "kid brother," Charles Hissey and his wife, Grace, and constant financial worries. Between April and July, John also asked her numerous times to ship him costumes and other paraphernalia for his shows, supplies his Captain apparently was unwilling or unable to procure. To make matters worse, during John's hospitalization, their beloved dog, "Mr. Dinkle," died.

After John was discharged, he returned to Columbus, Ohio. "I had been told to take a six months period of absolute rest," he later wrote, but "Two days after my arrival home [I] went to work at WBNS, Columbus." Their stay in Columbus was to be short-lived, however. As John related it:

> In February [1944], Beatrice Kay,[1] who has been a friend for several years, was playing the Palace in Columbus. She and her swell husband, Sylvan, had never heard my work. When they did hear me they insisted we had to come to New York. We sold the car, used that money for the gamble, and [moved to New York] to see what we could do.

---

[1] Born as Hannah Beatrice Kuper in 1907, Beatrice Kay performed as "Honey Kuper" and "Honey Day" for part of her career in Vaudeville, radio, motion pictures, sound recordings, night clubs, and television. A singer with a "whiskey" voice, she went on to becoming a headliner at Billy Rose's famed Diamond Horseshoe Nightclub in New York. She was on Mercury Theatre (directed by Orson Welles), and eventually hosted a radio show, *The Beatrice Kay Show.* She appeared at top nightclubs including San Francisco's austere Fairmont Hotel Venetian Room, the Moulin Rouge in Paris, Hollywood's famed Ciro's in Los Angeles, and at the El Rancho Hotel in Las Vegas. She also recorded several phonograph albums, and appeared in a 1945 motion picture about the club where she had performed in her earlier years—*Billy Rose's Diamond Horseshoe* (the film starred Betty Grable and Dick Haymes).

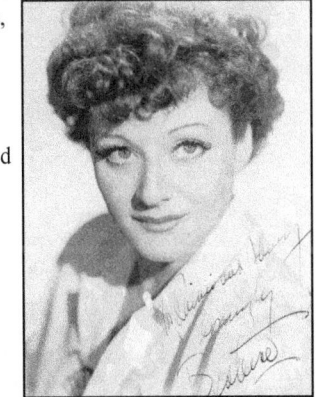

John, Rainie, Beatrice and her husband remained friends through the 1950s when Kay moved from New York to California.

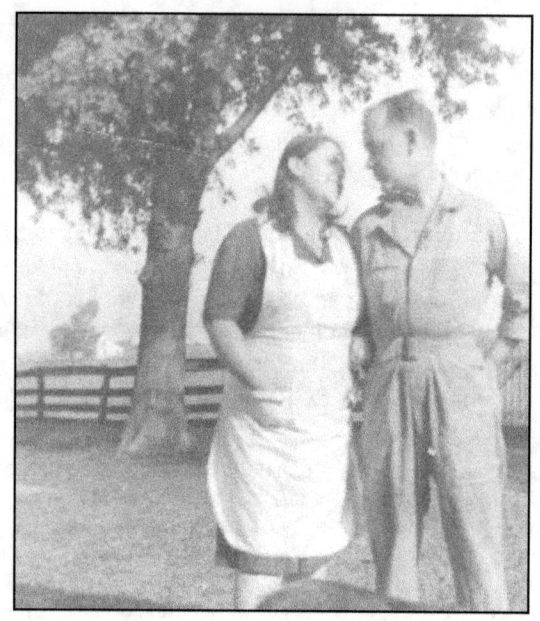

John and Rainie, September 1943, in Ohio.

No Business Like Show Business

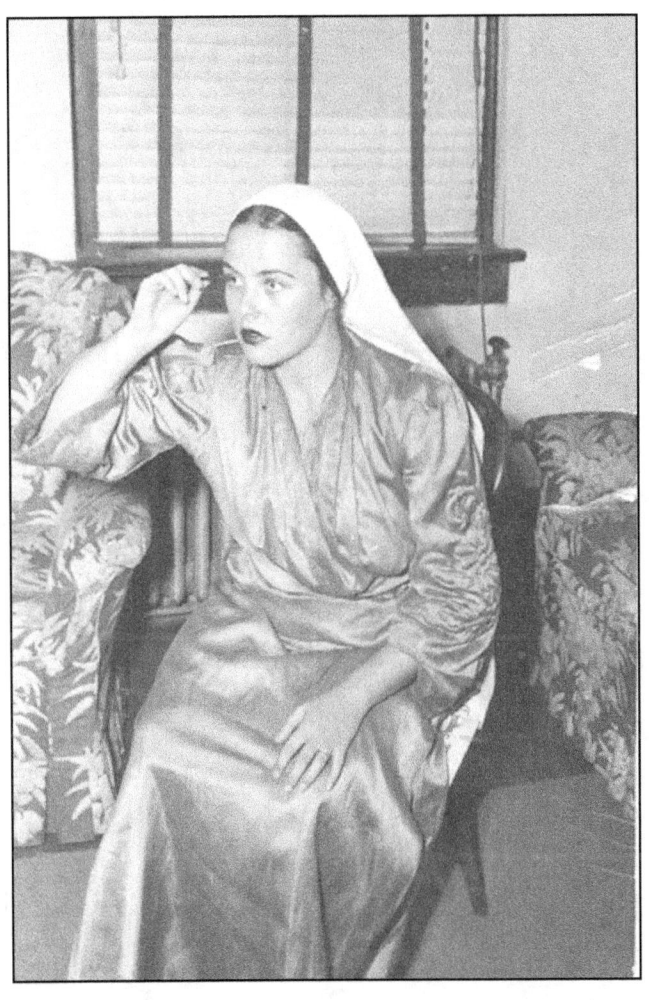

Previous page: Rainie Clarke applying stage makeup, date unknown.

Rainie and John packed up their meager belongings and struck out to make their way in the Big Apple. They met more initial success than many aspiring entertainers who hit the big city with big dreams. In 1945, a year after making the move to New York, John wrote his friends:

My first day I got lined up to audition to replace Ralph Edwards on *Truth or Consequences* [then a radio show]. Ralph was headed for the Army. Incidentally I was still in the last six running when Harry Von Zell won the thing. However Ralph didn't go. While that was still in the fire I auditioned at Columbia Broadcasting System [CBS] and was hired as a staff announcer. Got along very well there altho[ugh] there was very little money in it. I started to get some good shows like *People's Platform* and other serious shows. They were grooming me for a newscaster and I had several coast-to-coast newscasts each week. [Coast-to-coast broadcasting was still a relatively new phenomenon in 1944.] Was at CBS till June. Then I was offered a much better, much easier and much more lucrative position with William Esty and Company.[1]

For about a year and a half, John worked for Esty, producing a popular radio program called *Blind Date*, another program called *Thanks to the Yanks*, and was assistant director/producer for *Mystery in the Air*, a 13-week replacement show for *Abbot and*

---

[1] William Esty & Co. opened April 1, 1932, in New York, after Esty left the famous J. Walter Thompson advertising agency to strike out on his own. That November the agency won R.J. Reynolds Tobacco Co.'s Camel cigarettes and Prince Albert tobacco accounts. By the 1950s, its advertising campaign had made Camels the number one brand of cigarettes. The agency added the company's Winston in 1954 and Salem in 1956, as well as Cavalier, Doral and other brands. By 1945, Esty was the No. 21 agency in the U.S., relying mainly on RJR for about half of its $14 million in billings. Thanks to postwar ad spending, the agency broke into the top 10 in agency rankings, with billings of $27 million. Much of this growth was attributed to Colgate-Palmolive-Peet's Vel account, which was expanding into related soap product categories. Esty was later bought out several times and is now part of the Minneapolis-based Campbell-Mithun-Esty. Esty figured prominently in the 1980s suits against the tobacco industry for hiding knowledge of the ill effects on health of smoking.

Costello. He also handled the script, commercials, and contacts for the Hollywood-produced show, *Blondie*, and supervised a Minneapolis-originated show called *Quiz of the Twin Cities.*

John and Rainie lived on 61st Street in New York City, frequently entertaining guests and making show business contacts. As a youth, I heard several amusing stories about such entertaining, though it is unclear to me exactly when they occurred. Two that seem to be related to the immediate post-War period in New York—or possibly during the very early stages of the Korean War—when rationing was still in effect, were particularly memorable.

In one instance, John and Rainie bragged—and this, I suspect took place in Columbus, Georgia before John joined the Army—that they were able to amaze their dinner guests by providing dinners with ample servings of beef and other meat despite the strict rationing that should have precluded such abundance. They never tipped off their guests that in one instance, the tasty viand was rattlesnake, while several times they served big, juicy buffalo steaks, neither subject to rationing coupons. So delighted to eat their fill of meat, their guests never seemed to have noticed, and certainly didn't complain.

Once in New York, John and Rainie invited several friends over for dinner. Apparently everyone had enjoyed a lengthy cocktail "hour" (more likely several hours) as the hosts prepared a roast chicken. Apparently the bird was taking considerably longer than expected, and by the time John and Rainie got around to preparing to serve dinner, everyone was feeling very happy. John, ever the consummate host and a fine cook, decided *he* would put the finishing touches on the bird. He added a bit of flour to the juices to make a nice gravy, but found it too thick. So he added some water. Oops, now too thin. So, some more flour. Over-did it. Need some more water (and perhaps another drink). This cycle was repeated several times until John was satisfied and the poor, lonely chicken was virtually floating in a sea of gravy. Everyone laughed uproariously, and apparently all were too well oiled to really care that there was far more weak gravy than needed for one roaster.

By 1946, however, the gravy days were at least temporarily over. John lost his job at Esty and was "at liberty," working freelance jobs while he and Rainie were trying to raise their growing family (October, born in 1946; Christopher in 1949; and John Timothy in 1951) in an increasingly too small two-and-a-half room apartment. Money was very tight, especially since their first child—daughter October—was born the same year that John lost his position.

Over the next several years, John picked up work where he could, scraping together a living doing commercials, narration, ad hoc production and announcing, and temporary or fill-in announcing. In 1946, for example, he did a series of 15-minute transcribed dramatic shows on juvenile delinquency for the State of New York, narrated a series of television shows sponsored by Rittenhouse Chimes, a company that produced door chimes and other equipment and that had been a significant wartime industrial supplier to the U.S. Government.

Around 1948, John landed a job at New York's WINS radio,[2] where he hosted a four-hour-per-day disc-jockey show called *Going to Town* and received a *Billboard Magazine* award for his youth-oriented program called *Three Corner Club*. John was featured on the cover of the June 26, 1948 issue of the entertainment magazine, *Gotham Life: The Official Metropolitan Guide*. In the very early 1950's, John worked with the famous Osa Johnson—wife of the legendary pair of adventure and wildlife photography pioneers, Martin and Osa Johnson—to produce a 26-week series of half-hour films on ABC TV.[3]

Before long, however, he had moved to Newark, New Jersey's WNJR where he hosted *The Johnny Clarke Show*, a three-hour

---

[2.] After the company changed hands in 1953, it switched its programming to the new rock-and-roll, hiring the controversial Cleveland disc-jockey Alan Freed and Murray "The K" Kaufman.

[3.] The Johnsons pioneered the use of in-the-wild photography in places ranging from Borneo to Africa between 1917-1936 and produced dozens of movies shown in theaters across America. Martin was killed in a plane crash in 1937 in which Osa was badly injured. After recovering, she pioneered the genre of wildlife education programming on television with the show *Big Game Hunt*, which John narrated, eight years before Mutual of Omaha and Marlin Perkins introduced their popular series, *Wild Kingdom*. Osa also was one of the first to introduce a line of popular clothing modeled on the attire she use during her adventures. She died of a heart attack in 1953.

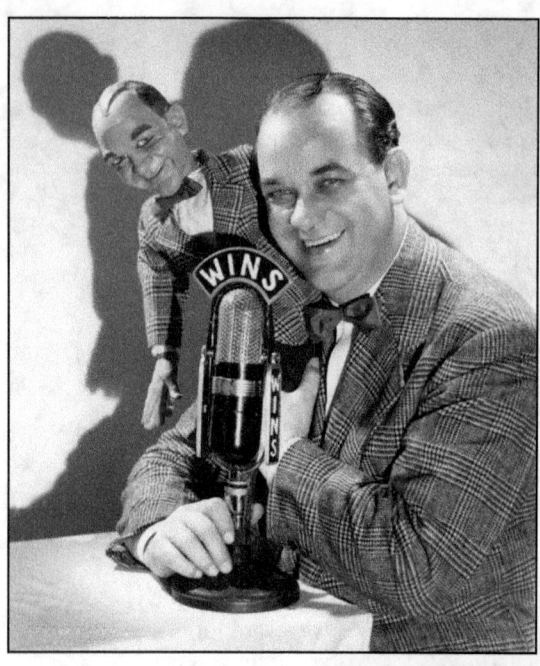

John Clarke's early radio years in New York.

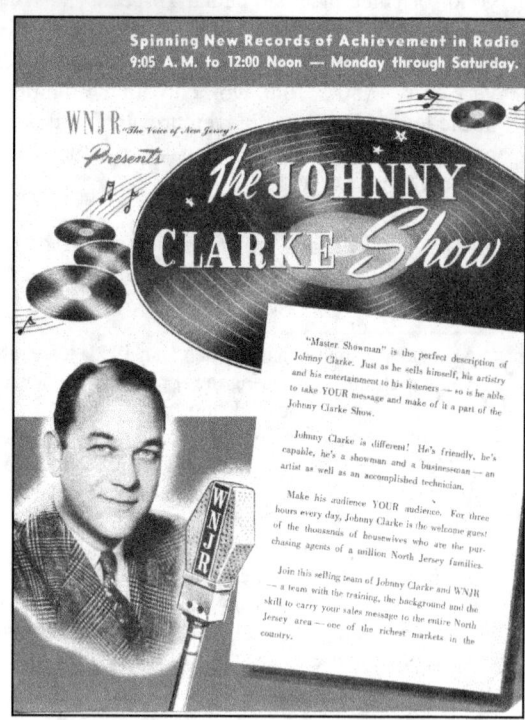

50

daily show of music and interviews and *Clarke's Clambake*, a two-hour Saturday teenage show. Despite the shows' popularity, Clarke's stay at each station appeared to be short, apparently the result of rapidly changing radio tastes and a series of six-month or one-year contracts.

John's next contract was with WCAU, a Philadelphia affiliate of CBS, for which he hosted a popular celebrity interview program called *The Steel Pier Show*, which featured discussions with famous personalities appearing at Atlantic City, New Jersey's various hot spots.

Despite these numerous radio, commercial, narration, acting, and producing jobs, work was sporadic and money remained tight. Rainie had taken a hiatus from working in entertainment. After arriving in New York, she later recalled with her typical sense of humor:

> I spent six months learning the beauty business (a revolting process which eventually turned my stomach). I gave this up and turned to exclusive millinery, getting a job in the workrooms of one of our notable male milliners (a revolting creature who eventually turned my stomach).

> My next five years of stomach-turning produced better results. I delivered three beautiful children who are much smarter than I am and therefore give me a rough go of it. These five years of domestic bliss were interrupted only once for a stint in TV as the voice of Elsie, the Borden cow. Under the circumstances, I naturally assumed that this was type casting.

A later publicity release explained: "Her 'Christopher' and Elsie's 'Beauregard' brought about a temporary retirement."[4] Apparently she took this job partly to supplement the family income. In one of the short stories she seems to have hoped to have published, Rainie later wrote a wonderful and moving account of this difficult time, apparently during the Christmas season of 1950.

[4.] The Christopher referred to here is the author.

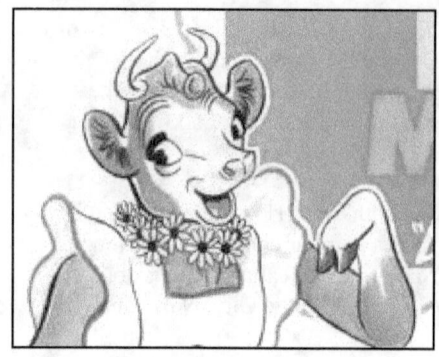

Elsie the Borden Cow

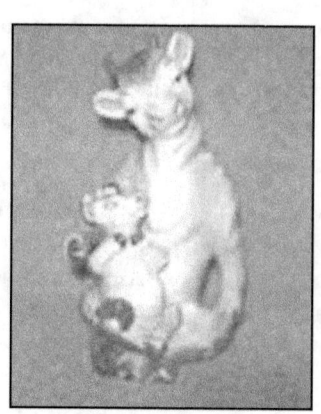

Elsie and Beauregard

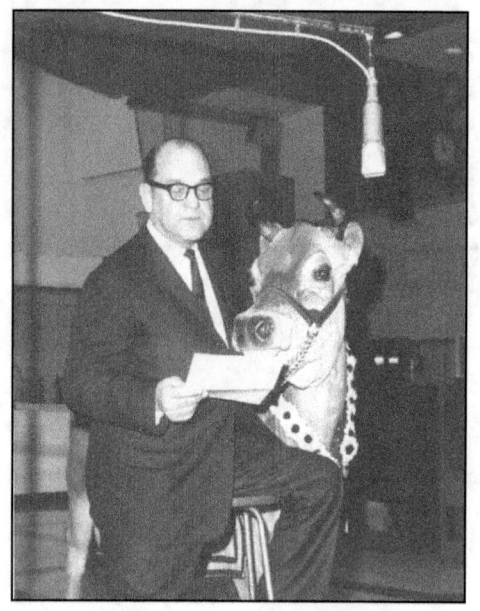

John with the "real" Elsie the Borden Cow.

Turkey and Trimmings
by
Rainie Clarke

My husband, John, reached forward and brushed the last stroke of white paint on the little stove. He stuck the brush in a can, took out a cigarette and lit it. Then, with his back against the wall, he exhaled and said, "How does it look?" I glanced up from the sewing machine.

"Oh, it's darling."

"Do you think Toby will like it?"

"She'll be ecstatic. I wish mine were half as nice"

"The refrigerator's cute too, huh?"

"It's marvelous. Santa Claus couldn't have done better." "

"Yes, but Santa's kitchens are made of metal. Toby says so."

"Well, that point is settled. I explained to her that Uncle Sam needs all the metal for planes in Korea. She's reconciled to a wooden kitchen." John got up and stretched.

"The refrigerator looks pretty authentic," he said, "but I wish I hadn't spent our last two dollars for the handle. Now we *will* have to open the piggy-bank for groceries. My unemployment check doesn't arrive until Tuesday."

"That won't help us over Christmas."

"No. I know it."

"Well, never mind, honey. We'll make out somehow." I sighed. Being "at liberty", a familiar pattern of show-business, had reared its ugly head again. It had been going on since late September when John's summer broadcasts had ended. So far we had kept afloat, but just squeezing by from one unemployment check to another was a belt-tightening process that was beginning to gall.

As I yawned and lit a cigarette, John called from the tiny kitchenette, "Want a cup of coffee?" "Yes," I answered. Then, with elaborate unconcern, I said, "How did things go today?"

"Just about the same," he answered. "I must have been to a dozen advertising agencies. I stopped in at NBC -- stopped at a couple of independent stations. Same reaction every place. Oh...you know what Christmas week is like." "

Don't get discouraged, honey," I said, trying to sound

more optimistic than I felt. "Things always pick up after the first of the year."

John brought in the coffee. He handed me my cup and sat on the arm of the couch sipping his. "I feel guilty that I'm not writing letters and answering ads tonight, though," he said.

"Is there any place left that you haven't already written?" I asked him. Then I added, "Forget it for awhile. Nobody's going to notice his mail this week anyway. How do you like Toby's doll?" I handed him the drum majorette I had just finished dressing. "She's great," he said. "Do you think Toby will recognize her?"

John answered, "No. The new wig makes her look entirely different. If Toby doesn't see the broken toes, you're all set." I leaned forward and began to stitch. "Oh, she won't," I said. "I glued on these boots to make sure of that. What else do we still have to do?"

John checked off the list. "The stove and refrigerator are finished... and the doll?" "Finished," I nodded. "Let's see,' said John, "I still have to give Chris' little sled a coat of red paint -- I guess that's all." He took another gulp of coffee and said, "You must know I feel like a heel not having anything for you." "Oh, sweetheart, I don't have anything; for you, either," I lied. I had knitted him a pair of socks.

We finished our coffee and John carried our cups to the kitchen. He washed and dried them. The kitchen was too small to leave even two cups and saucers sitting in the way.

"I think I'll have these pajamas finished for Chris' doll by the time you get that coat of paint on. That should just about wind things up."

John stroked paint ever the toy sled. "If you're finished first," he said, "will you get the piggy-bank? I'll open it while I still have the tools out."

I folded the sewing machine and put it away. Then I picked up the remnant box and tidied the floor, making sure to remove all evidence of Mrs. Santa Claus' activities. I tiptoed through the children's room and returned in a minute with a colorful papier mache pig which we had been feeding with change all year.

"He feels pretty fat," I said. "Maybe we can afford a small turkey."

"Maybe," John maybied, "but don't forget, we also need a

tree, and groceries for over the week-end."

"Let's see the patient," said John. I handed him the pig and he shook it vigorously. "No good," he said, shaking his head. "We'll have to operate. Scalpel."

I handed him the saw.

"Retractor!"

I handed him the hammer. He grinned up at me.

"I guess this is what is known as 'bringing home the bacon'."

I laughed, but not as heartily as I might have, for he was pouring out the contents of Pig and, as far as I could see, there were too many pennies.

The contents totaled $8.13.

"Well," John said, "there's the loot." And after a pause, "I guess it's groceries *and* turkey, or groceries *and* tree, but it can't be all three." "No," I agreed. What'll it be?" he asked. I mused, "The children will be so excited they won't notice what they're eating."

"You're right."

"There's no way we can 'fake' a tree, is there?"

"No."

"Then there's the answer. Groceries and *tree*. I'll make a meat loaf. I guess that's that!"

"Yeah," John said wryly, "I guess that's that!"

On Christmas eve, John and Toby bundled up against the weather and set out on their quest for our Christmas tree. It was early evening and I heard a neighboring record player blaring out "Jingle Bells". I set the sugar bowl on the table and glanced out of the large window facing uptown. It was already dark and the neon signs were winking on both sides of Broadway up to 73rd street. Chris sat in his crib in the next room and mumbled syllables to me. He was engrossed in ripping- pages from an old magazine and I was too discouraged to suggest a mere constructive activity.

That $8.13 wasn't going to spread very far.

"Iggle ells," said Chris.

"Yes, 'Jingle Bells'," I answered.

I turned my back on the view, the only redeeming feature of our two and a half room apartment. Slowly I walked back to the kitchen.

"Kitchen!'" I snorted. "Humph: Broom closet is more like

it. Everything piled on top of everything else...why, I couldn't even let Toby help me with the Christmas cookies because there isn't room in this hole for two of us at the same time!"

Resentment and hostility began to well up inside me and I flung open the door to the refrigerator. "Well," I thought, "at least I won't have to worry abut what to fix for supper! Here we go again! Hamburger! ...honestly, I could write a cookbook on seven hundred different ways to prepare hamburger! " Hot tears slid down my cheeks and bounced off my chin. "The real problem," I muttered, "is how I'm going to make two pounds of hamburger look like a Christmas turkey tomorrow!" I busied myself patting the ground meat into little rounds. Mechanically I went about opening cans of vegetables and slicing home-made bread as I silently damned the vagaries of show-business.

The radio mumbled Christmas commercials, intermingled with carols and, with brightening spirits, I began to enumerate the last minute things still to be accomplished. "When John and Toby get home with the tree, we'll eat supper...then hang the stockings... then read "The Night Before Christmas" . . . tuck the children into bed...prayers ... and then," I sighed, "The work begins. My, it's taking them a long time to buy that tree." I laid the meat patties in the skillet. "Meanwhile" I muttered, "how am I going to make two pounds of hamburger look like a turkey tomorrow? Well, old girl, it could be worse. Suppose you didn't have any hamburger... there must be lot of people who don't... now if you stretch the meat loaf with macaroni. . . and then, perhaps you could splurge and put two hard-boiled eggs in the center... just to surprise the children when it's sliced.. ...then maybe you could shape it like a bird...No. Better just make it plain and decorate the top...a sprig of holly just before it's served?...."

At that moment the phone rang. I wiped my hands on a tea towel and picked up the receiver. It was the desk clerk of our apartment-hotel. "There's a large package down here for you people. Do you want me to send it up?" "Yes, thank you," I replied, wondering what it could possibly be. Almost immediately the door bell rang and I opened the door. The elevator operator placed a large cardboard carton on the chair next to the door.

"Merry Christmas," he said and disappeared. Excitement pulsed through me and I tingled from head to foot, for on the end of the carton, printed in large type, were the words "CATSKILL

SMOKED TURKEY", and in smaller letters, the caution to "refrigerate immediately".

As I glanced at the gift card I prayerfully murmured., "Thank God, heaven, providence and good friends," and started tearing open the package, layer by layer, marveling the whole time at the care and precision of the wrapping;. I slid the magnificent bird out of his insulated bag:, left the papers and boxes in the chair and carried the turkey to the kitchen. I had just started to rearrange the refrigerator to accommodate the gift when the door bell sounded. I rushed to the door and threw it wide to a merry daughter and a glowing husband, both exhilarated from their walk in the brisk cold. Happiness shone in both their faces as they dragged the tree into the foyer.

John set a paper shopping bag on top of the wrappings. "Don't touch that," he said, pointing to the bag. Toby danced up and down, echoing her daddy. "Don't touch it, Mommy! Don't touch it! It's a secret!" she shouted. I was too elated about the turkey to pay much attention.

John set the tree in the corner, saying, "It looks like a pretty good Christmas. We got a beautiful tree. It cost less than I expected. It's really better to wait until Christmas eve. Dealers don't want to be stuck with a surplus of trees and you can buy them cheaper."

"Yes, dear, that's fine. Wonderful," I interrupted, "but come in the kitchen and see the surprise." I half dragged him with me and proudly displayed the turkey. "And just *look* at the way this thing was packaged!" I said, as I rushed across the floor to show him what I considered to be a fine example of modern mailing ingenuity. As I reached into the melee to extract the gift card, I dislodged the shopping bag. It teetered precariously. Then it toppled ever and hit the floor.

CRASH!

Complete silence. My stomach did a half-gainer. Both of us stood rooted to the floor. Even the usually irrepressible Toby stared mutely at the fallen bag which obviously contained a debacle.

Suddenly, without a word, John wheeled, walked swiftly through the children's room into the bathroom and closed the door firmly behind him.

Crushed, frightened, I turned back to the kitchen and automatically set about finishing dinner. As I made the frequent trips to and from the table, I carefully avoided glancing at the accusing sight of the paper bag still laying on the floor. Somehow I couldn't bear to pick it up.

I settled the children at the table, tied on Chris' bib and sat down in my accustomed place. Cautiously, Toby ran a chubby finger along the edge of the table. Finally she said, "Mommy, what's the matter with Daddy?" "I don't know, darling. Just be quiet and wait."

John walked into the room, sat down and spread the napkin across his lap. We said Grace. Silently he served the plates. Without much enthusiasm, we started to eat. "What's the matter, Daddy?" Toby said. I shushed her. "But I want to know what's wrong," she insisted. "Toby, you will please eat your dinner!" I said firmly.

John sighed and looked across the table at me. His eyes were suspiciously moist. Finally he said, "Well, honey, I guess you might as well know. I've been saving carfare for a month to buy you that milk glass apothecary jar you wanted. I bought it tonight while we were out. That is what just smashed into a thousand fragments . I'm sorry, sweetheart. I can't afford to get you anything else. That was your only Christmas present." His voice broke. I never felt more miserable.

We finished dinner. I undressed the children and read them their story. We heard their prayers, kissed them and tucked them in for the night.

I had cleared the table, washed the dishes and was standing at the front window gazing up Broadway when John came in from the back hall with the ladder and the box of decorations. He set them down and joined me at the window. Traffic signals were shimmering like strips of tree lights. Last minute shoppers were scurrying up and down the street. The peaceful Christmas eve quiet that prevails, even in busy Manhattan, hovered over everything.

As John put his arms around me, the new baby stirred and rolled over. Afraid of breaking the spell, I whispered, "This Christmas Eve has been worth more to me than all the milk glass jars in the world. It's a present I'll remember for the rest of my life."

> John kissed the drying tears on my face. As if by silent mutual consent, we walked across the room, picked up the mutilated little package and placed it under the barren tree. We stood and looked at it for a minute.
>
> "You know, we're really very lucky," said John. "We have each other and the children...and we're soon going to add another member to the family....Come on, honey. Let's un-pack the trimmings. We have a lot of work to do!"

Apparently in 1951, John landed his first relatively permanent and steady radio job, albeit in the form of a long stretch of summer replacement positions and special assignments at WOR radio and television in New York.

> WOR signed on February 22, 1922, with the help of engineers Orville Orvis and Jack Poppele, who powered up a DeForest transmitter on the 6th floor of Bamberger's Department Store at 131 Market St. in Newark and played Al Jolson's record of "April Showers." ...In 1949, WOR started a sister TV station, WOR-TV, on channel 9...In December 1952, the Bamberger Broadcasting Service transferred WOR to General TeleRadio, a subsidiary of the General Tire and Rubber Company, and when General Tire acquired RKO, the corporate name became RKO-General. In 1956, WOR created "Music From Studio X". It was simply continuous pop music, but it originated from a special high-fidelity studio and each clean new record was touched by a needle only one time.[5]

Some of the most famous radio, and later TV, personalities got their start or worked at WOR, including John B. Gambling, John A. Gambling, and John R. Gambling, three generations of the same family who continuously hosted *Rambling with Gambling* from 1924-2008; Ed & Pegeen ("Peggy") Fitzgerald, Arlene Francis, Patricia McCann, Long John Nebel, Bernard Meltzer, Barry Farber, Jean Shepherd, Bob & Ray, Jack O'Brian, Bob Grant and Gene Klavin; Dorothy Kilgallen and her husband Dick Kollmar; Mary

---

[5] http://www.wor710.com/pages/58403.php and http://en.wikipedia.org/wiki/WOR_(AM).

Margaret McBride; Dennis Miller (from an outside syndicator); Bill O'Reilly (from an outside syndicator); Joan Rivers; and currently Glenn Beck and Lou Dobbs.

John worked for WOR for six years doing special assignments on TV, including as staff announcer for such programs as *The Merry Mailman* and *Million Dollar Movie* and for four years, served as a 26-week summer replacement for staff announcers and in other assignments.

With finances apparently now stabilized, in Rainie's words:

> In the spring of 1953 when we were finally convinced that two and a half rooms would not accommodate five outsize people, we bought a house. On September 1, 1953, we moved into the house.

And therein lies another tale.

Happy Daze
By
Rainie Clarke

For a full scale Donnybrook Fair, I will give top billing to moving day every time. August 30th [1953] was no exception. John had to work and I was left to organize the moving. I considered myself lucky that I had only one child and two dogs to impede the march of progress. The apartment hotel where we had made our home for nine years was of the gay [18]90's era. It had had its face lifted several times, and in more recent days had undergone several bouts of major surgery.

However, it still retained features of its original self, one of which was the freight elevator. This was used not only for freight, but to transport linen, mops, buckets, maids, and general paraphernalia. The management refused us the use of it until after 11 am. So the moving men, who had arrived promptly at 9 o'clock, spent the first two hours carting things out the front door, and piling them in the hall. As the maids and their equipment were always dispersed to their various floors no later than 9:30, this was just another example of our landlord's obstructionist policies.

Shortly after eleven, the more burly of the two men, who claimed to have been a dockwalloper at one time, rebelled. "Give me five minutes to get this thing straightened out," he said, and disappeared into the passenger car. He refused to say exactly what transpired, but he returned within the allotted time wearing a "We-have-met-the-enemy-and- he-is-ours" look, and we had no more trouble with the management.

Our apartment exhibited its own brand of scar tissue in the form of holes in closet walls, shelves built into ancient door-ways, and a dimly lit back hall, almost too narrow for passage. As the family increased and space diminished, Pappy [Rainie's life-long affectionate nickname for John] had ingeniously converted every inch of available area into shelves and closets for storage. Every clothes closet had at least one chest of drawers in it. Some had two. Every doorway except the front one had shelves built over and around it. Even a hole in the pantry wall had been filled with orange crate shelving. The result was that, as the moving men carried down one load to put in the van, I was dragging things out from all the these hidden crevices, giving a kind of Sorcerer's Ap-prentice atmosphere to the whole proceeding.

At one-thirty, Mr. Burly came in the door mopping his brow. "Lady," he said, "I dunno where it's all coming from, but the next time I come home from a vacation, I'm gonna call on you to do my packing!" Then he added, "Where's the telephone? I gotta call the office for another van."

By three-thirty the last items were loaded. I strapped Timmy in the baby seat and drove out to the house, arriving about twenty minutes ahead of the furniture. Timmy played contentedly in a play-pen in the back yard while I directed traffic from the front porch. The job was completed by seven o'clock. I figured the cost (10 hours at $12 an hour) was pretty reasonable considering what we had accomplished. But as I drove back to the city I reflected that the Burly Dray and Haulage Co. would probably case the job on every two-and-a-half room [job] from that day on.

*   *   *

When we operate on logic, we practically always wind up in a mess. When we follow [Pappy's] hunches, we rarely make a mistake. I must admit, however, that it has taken me 15 years to build up enough confidence in this system so that I only argue on about one out of five decisions.

We once bought a Buick, a convertible sedan far beyond our means. John's employer tried to talk us out of it on the theory that we were young and inexperienced. He argued that "It was not the initial expense. It was the upkeep." We bought it anyway. Two years later, before we moved to New York, we sold it for $295 more than we had paid. Mr. Employer is still shaking his head and we are still operating for the most part, on hunch.

Toby and Chris returned from camp on Saturday before labor Day. Toby entered school the following Thursday. The next Monday morning she came downstairs for breakfast, complaining that she didn't feel very well. We took one glance at her face. It was puffed up like a melon. John said, "My God, the mumps!" I sent her back to bed and called the doctor.

"Nothing to do but keep her in bed. She'll be alright in a week," he told me. He added, "You'll have to notify the Board of Health, though."

I called the Board of Health and they sent an inspector to see us. He was a dear little man who looked like Happy in Snow White and the Seven Dwarfs. Mr. Happy told me that Toby would be alright, but added, "Mrs. Clarke, have you or your husband ever had the mumps?" I said that John had, but I had not. He warned me, "Then you must be very careful. Mumps can be extremely serious for an adult."

If there is anything calculated to make an adult feel asinine, it is contracting a childhood disease. One afternoon about 10 days later, John and I were back in the woods using a cross-cut saw to cut up an old black cherry log that had fallen across the path. I

62

was tired when we finished the job, so I went up to the house to bathe before starting dinner. As I glanced in the mirror, I discovered the left side of my face swollen like bread dough. The next morning, Chris's face was swollen too. I called the Board of Health and Mr. Happy paid us another visit. He advised me to go to bed, but failing that, he confined me to the property for fourteen days. This was the second time we had been quarantined in less than two months.

* * *

Autumn began to finger-paint the woods, and the weeds on the back hill shriveled like cheap bacon...

Black locusts have a peculiar beauty unlike any other tree. Our property abounds in them. They tower some 60 to 80 feet into the air. In winter they look like gaunt old skeletons. In spring, they develop clusters of white blossoms, something like wisteria, which they shed in a gentle May-time snow. In summer they burst into sporadic clouds of lacy green fringe, and sway gracefully in the wind, creaking like old rocking chairs.

The maple leaves were beginning to burn themselves crisp when a large moving van arrived one day from Ohio. As they began to unload, I was beside myself with excitement. It was just like Christmas: until we started unpacking trunks and cartons. I wonder how many tears have been shed over needless ruin caused by negligent storage companies? I wept my share of them as I removed layer after layer of my mother's beautiful table linen, John's mother's hand embroidered sheets and pillow cases, rotted woolen blankets, and water stained satin draperies, all reeking of mildew. The carnage was a crushing blow. And the climax was two missing barrels containing our best china, all of our glasses, and a great deal of silverware. The storage firm and the moving company are still passing the buck on this deal.

Every piece of furniture had to be vacuumed, scrubbed, shampooed, and polished before it could be brought into the house. I set out to salvage what linen and draperies I could. For three weeks, my 200 foot clothesline was full, morning to night, seven days a week. The front lawn was dotted with table cloths and curtain stretchers.

I tried every bleaching method I had ever heard of and came up with a few ideas of my own. My reputation as a laundress exceeded even that of my neighbor, Mary Mullowney, who had four children, three of them in diapers.

Every night as soon as the dishes were washed, I ironed until bedtime. One night 65 of my mother's linen hand towels rolled through the ironer like a great ribbon of toothpaste. I believe this holds the record for wasted effort as not more than a half dozen have been used from that day to this.

Gradually the days were becoming more winey. One night in early October, John called everybody into the living room. "We're going to have our first fire," he said. The children "Oohed" and "Aaahed," settling to the floor like autumn leaves. Pappy struck a match, leaned forward and lit it. The kindling caught, then the locust log. Suddenly flames billowed, licking at the bricks and the mantle. I gasped, the children shrieked, and the beautiful white porcelain paint turned to black porcelain blisters before our eyes.

With great presence of mind, Pappy doused the fire quickly, and then investigated. Almost immediately, he discovered the trouble. Instead of opening the flue, he had closed it. The mantle has since been sanded and repainted, but even under the best circumstances, white bricks have a disgusting habit of becoming pink bricks after the third or fourth fire. No more white brick mantles for me. If we ever build a house, no more white woodwork either. I'm going to have everything painted battleship grey and keep it that way until Timmy is 35 years old.

Rainie later wrote about the joys of their new suburban life.

Suburban Pleasures

City-bred people are funny. Any amount of taxi horns, clanging fire engines, swearing truck drivers, gunning motors, back-fires or ambulance sirens react on them as a lullaby; but without exception, every city dweller who visited us has issued the same complaint when we enquired how he slept. "I'd have been fine except for the goddam birds!" I don't feel that way. I love hearing the birds at any time, but especially early in the morning.

We enjoyed the fall. Frequently we would sit in the back yard for a cigarette between jobs. The Virginia Creeper blazed crimson trails up the trunks of the black cherry trees. Maples were turning alternately yellow and red, while the locusts retained enough of a green backdrop to point up the rainbow colors. The woods looked as if it had been painted with a palette knife, while underfoot the carpet of leaves rustled like taffeta. We followed the activities of industrious squirrels and chipmunks as we discussed our plans for the house.

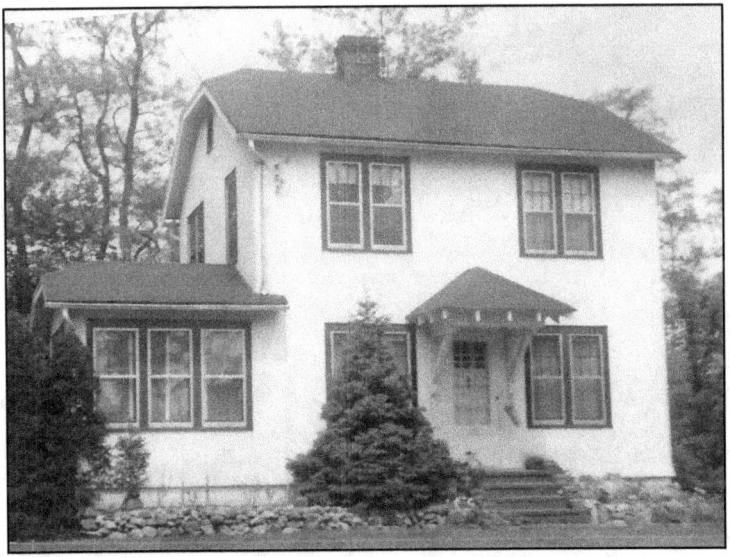

174 Mountain Ave., Ridgewood, New Jersey in the late 1950s.
The sunporch on the left was Rainie's room.

65

In the Lap of God

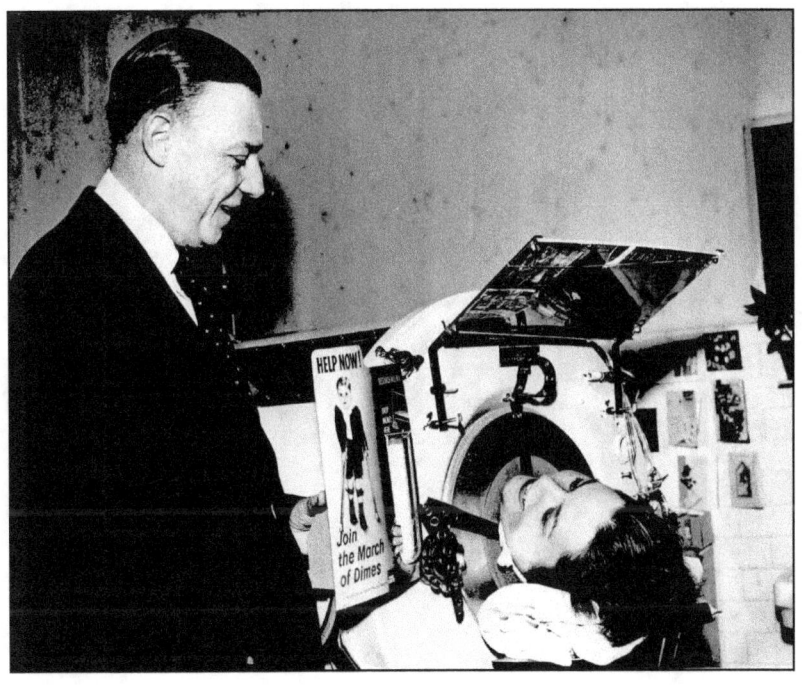

Previous page: "March of Dimes" publicity photo of Rainie in an iron lung at Bergen Pines Hospital, Bergen County, New Jersey, during the winter of 1953-1954.

The Clarkes' suburban idyll of a house, yard with picket fence, three kids, two dogs and a normal life was about to come to a crashing end, however. On October 29, according to a later account by John:

> She felt tired and lazy with muscular aches and pains in her back...I insisted she see the Doctor... On Friday, October 30, she had a 3:00 pm appointment. Before Rainie went in for examination I said to the doctor, "Go over her thoroughly for polio, will you?" When Rainie came out to the car she said, "The Doctor told me what you said to him and says you can relax. He gave me a severe examination and finds no trace [of polio]. However he finds I am tired and a little anemic and gave me prescriptions: one for that, and one for sleeping tonight and tomorrow night and wants me to stay in bed and rest a couple of days.

Rainie failed to rest—with three small children, one recovering from the mumps, and a new house to put in order, who could blame her?—and became more run down.

She later told the story in her own inimitable way:

In the Lap of God
By
Rainie Clarke

Friday [October 30, 1953] I awoke to a caucus of blue jays; stretched, rolled over and contemplated the scarlet Virginia Creeper through the hall window. It was a moment of pure privacy, rare in a family of five, and I guarded it jealously. Gradually I became aware of a tremendous sense of fatigue. I reviewed the end of the previous day, searching for the fasteners on which to hang my morning. Hazily I recalled John's having muttered something about walking down to the big brook. I glanced at his bed. It was rumpled and he was gone. Then I smelled the coffee. "Come on, old girl," I whispered, "It's later than you think." Slowly I pulled my legs out from under the covers and dropped them over the side of the bed. For a minute I considered crawling back in, but force of

---

habit is strong. I threw on slacks, a sweat-shirt, and my gunboats and went down to the kitchen.

"Good afternoon, sleepyhead," John laughed. "Have a cup of coffee?" I reached for the cup.

"Where's Toby?"

"Gone to school."

"Is it that late?" I studied the coffee. The cup looked heavy.

"Are you ready for the hike?" I asked?

"What hike?"

"Didn't you say you wanted to go down to the brook this morning?"

"No. But if you want to go, we will."

I was too tired to argue the point.

We wound our way down the hill, between the locusts, to the bridge. Crossing over, I looked down at Real Stream. It was weaving and swirling as I had never seen it before. "I must be dizzy." I thought. The feeling passed.

"You know, that place over there," John said, pointing to the right of the path, "would be ideal for a tennis court."

"Sounds expensive."

"Not if we do it ourselves. If we made it of black top, the children could ride their wheel toys on it. Then in the winter we could flush and freeze it for ice skating."

I shivered. John looked at me.

"If you'll pardon me for saying so, you look like hell this morning," he said.

70

"I'm beginning to feel like hell, too," I answered.

"Come on, let's go back up to the house," he suggested. "I don't think you ought to be roaming around the woods, the way you look."

We recrossed the bridge and started up the hill. I felt as though I were moving under water, like a deep sea diver, each leg weighted down with lead. It took controlled determination to set my feet, one in front of the other. We gained the top of the hill and walked around the house to the front yard. Mrs. Corbin was clipping the last of her chrysanthemums so we stood and chatted with her for a few minutes.

I excused myself and walked over to the car, sat in the front seat and lit a cigarette, shaking from head to foot. "This is ridiculous," I thought. "I'm going inside and lie down."

John shoved the thermometer at me. "Take your temperature," he said. I protested. "Take it, honey," he insisted. He leafed through the phone book. "There's a doctor over on Godwin Avenue. We've passed his shingle several times. I'm going to call him." He dialed the number, questioning me with his eyes. "It's 101," I told him.

I sank into a chair in the doctor's waiting: room. John held a whispered conference with him at the door.

"I'll wait in the car with the children," he called to me, and left.

As the doctor concluded his examination, I said, "What did Mr. Clarke ask you to do? Check for polio?"

"What makes you ask that?" he smiled.

"The test for reflexes you just performed."

He folded his arms and pushed the stethoscope into his cheek.

"What is the matter with me?" I asked.

"It's perfectly simple," he replied. "You've picked up a virus somewhere. But there's something else," he said, crossing over to his desk. "I think you're anemic." He started to write out a prescription.

My mouth flew open. "Anemic! I never realized anyone weighing 200 pounds could be anemic!"

"Oh, yes," he answered. "And that's another thing. You're going to have to take off some of that weight."

He handed me two prescriptions. "One of these is a sedative and the other a liver medicine. Go home and rest. I think you'll be alright in a couple of days."

As I stood in the closet, my head pressed against the wall, struggling for enough strength to change my clothes, I kept repeating, "I'll be alright in a couple of days. The doctor said so."

Finally I grabbed a housecoat and stumbled over to the bed. I called Toby, who was in her room playing with dolls. "Tell Daddy I'm lying down for a few minutes, honey. I'll be down in half an hour to start supper."

Oblivion . . . cloudy and grey ... and swirling . . . voices drifting up from somewhere ... voices and sounds ... and odors ....windows ... fading in and out.

I rolled over. The clock said 6:30. John was dressing. "Where are you going, honey?"

"I'm getting ready for work. How do you feel?"

"So-so. Confused...What ever happened to Saturday?"

"This is it."

"Oh."

I thought a long time.

"The children will be so disappointed. I promised to take them out for trick- or-treat."

"Mrs. Corbin said she would take them. Will you be alright if they're gone for an hour or two?"

"Sure."

"Call me at the station if you need me?"

"Sure."

"Goodbye, darling. I'll be home as soon as I can get back."

I slept. Then waked. Then dozed and waked again. The children were trooping up the stairs.

"Mother, we had so much fun."

"We brought you some treats."

"Look, Mommy, some treats."

"Can you dress yourselves for bed, children?"

"Yes, Mommy, but what about Timmy?"

"Bring his things in here to me."

I folded his diapers. "Climb up on top of these, Timmy."

Somehow I pinned the diapers and got his sleeper on him.

"Can you climb into your crib, sweetheart?"

"Yep."

"Then you children tell Mommy 'Goodnight' and go to bed."

The boys crawled up the bed to kiss me.

"G'nite, Mommy."

"G'nite, Mommy."

They pattered into their room.

"Do you feel any better, Mommy?"

"No, Toby, dear. Go to bed now."

"Can I help you?"

"If you can I'll call you. Good night, darling."

The hours dragged by. The hands on the clock seemed glued to its face. I struggled to the bathroom. Coming back, I thought, "Oh God, oh God! I'll never make it!"

I ricocheted from wall to wall. With one final spurt of effort, I fell across the foot of the bed...

The sun was pouring in the hall window, leaving a long exclamation point of light across the rug. I wondered idly, why the man was wearing light grey shoes in October. "It's not "October, though," I thought. "It's November. November 1st. As a matter of fact, it's All Saint's Day."

The doctor's voice sliced through my thoughts like a scalpel. "We'll have to have a spinal tap before I can tell." John and the doctor walked down the hall. "If I may use the phone, I'll call the county hospital for the ambulance." Both of them ran downstairs.

The stretcher couldn't make the turn in the hall. John came bounding up the steps with a straight chair. They tied me in it with a bathrobe cord and carried me down to the first floor. All the pieces began to fall apart.

Somewhere a siren sounded ... a mournful wail ascending to a high-pitched scream ...pierced by the dissonance of squealing tires. Doors .... elevators ... tile walls ... white walls .. .white dissolving into white ... white to white and unto white return ... pins and needles, needles and pins ... when a girl's married ... when a girl's married ... and needles and pins ... and... needles ... a voice in my head. "You must not move for eight hours ." . . . You must not move for eight hours ... You must not move ... You must not move ... You must not ... can't breathe ... must not ... can't breathe... can't breathe ... can't breathe ... can't BREATHE......

...

John stood in the hospital corridor. He watched the doctor walk slowly toward him.

"How do you do? Doctor Lenz?'" he asked.

The doctor smiled his "yes".

"My name is Clarke. How is my wife? "

"Mr. Clarke, it is a little too soon to tell. With polio we are never sure."

"Then it's definitely polio?"

"Oh, there was no question about that. Only what type."

"I see. And the type?"

Doctor Lenz pulled back his isolation gown and reached into his pocket for his glasses. "The lab report came back this morning, just after we put Mrs. Clarke in the respirator. The diagnosis is spinal-bulbar poliomylitis."

"Will she be able to walk again?"

Doctor Lenz sighed. "That is the first question you people always ask."

He pulled out a handkerchief to polish his lenses. "Right now, the question is, 'Will she be able to breathe?' ".

John spoke in the agony of frustration. "What can I do?"

"There is nothing you can do, Mr. Clarke. Get shots of gamma-globulin for your children. Outside of that, wait." He closed the interview.

Fourteen days of waiting. Fourteen days of quarantine. Fourteen days of milk bottles on the front curb, mail on the sidewalk, panic in the block.

On the fifteenth afternoon, John went to the hospital for his regular visit. His wife's special nurse greeted him. "Good afternoon, Mr. Clarke. We have good news for you today." She unlocked the 'lung' and pulled it out. "Your wife can breathe for three minutes on her own."

On the fifteenth night, John received a call from the hospital. "Mr. Clarke, this is Doctor Lenz. Come immediately. Your wife has had a relapse."

He sat in the reception room, chain-smoking. Occasionally the static sounds of the hospital were broken by the frightened cry of a child. He was aware of an undercurrent of sound. Thump, thump. Thump, thump. Thump, thump. "The respirators," he thought. He watched the big hospital clock in the hall. The seconds ticked off relentlessly, like dripping water. He lit a fresh cigarette and crushed the old one.

Quite suddenly, the door to his wife's room opened and Doctor Lenz was moving toward him with a deliberateness born of fatigue.

"Doctor Lenz?"

The doctor shook his head. "I've done everything I can for her." The doctor spread his fingers and studied his nails.

"All we can do now is leave her in the lap of God."

In a letter to friends and relatives shortly after Rainie was admitted to the hospital, John explained in more factual and much more sobering terms his recollection of events:

> Sunday, November 1, 9:30 am — Her leg was worse and she was sore all along her back and legs and couldn't rise or sit up in bed without being held. The Doctor came almost immediately, examined her thoroughly, called the hospital and ordered an ambulance. I followed them, got her admittance papers straightened out and hurried back to the youngsters who had played in the back yard under the eyes of the next door neighbors... I returned there about 3:00 pm and found they had run a spinal test and were reasonably sure it was polio although the head of the department wasn't there and they couldn't completely diagnose without his approval. Later Sunday evening it was confirmed.
>
> On Monday afternoon, the family doctor and the Health Officer arrived together, the doctor to give the youngsters Gamma Globulin, and the Health Officer to quarantine us to a very strict quarantine where we were not even allowed to mail a postcard or anything. Because of Rainie being on the critical list, and not being able to get *any help anywhere*, he did allow me to put the children in the car, roll the windows up tight, go directly to the hospital, leave the children in the car while I saw Rainie and come directly home.
>
> Monday, when I called at 7:00 am they said she had had some difficulty in breathing and it had been necessary to give her oxygen during the night. Around 11, they told me she had stopped breathing shortly after I had called and that it had been necessary to put her in a respirator. That afternoon, when I was allowed to see her (the doctor allowed me 5 minutes), she was reasonably bright although quite miserable in the Iron Lung (or respirator). She didn't change much during the whole week and seemed to be adapting herself to the lung pretty well.
>
> Sunday, the 8th, after one week in the hospital I had an op-

portunity for a long chat with the doctor, who said, "Mr. Clarke I don't mean to sound conceited, nor do I mean to be alarming but I think we should face facts. I've spent my whole life on polio both in Europe and here and I think I know about as much about it as anyone. I have the most competent staff would [sic. Probably "one"] can assemble and the best scientific equipment money can buy. I have seen many strange things with this disease. Both of Rainie's legs and her right arm are completely paralyzed as well as her breathing apparatus. I would say she'll be in the lung several months and it would be a matter of years for complete rehabilitation. I could be wrong. There are times when through sheer will-power and guts I am most pleasantly surprised in patients. Rainie has the will and I hope she'll be one of those patients."

Monday, Tuesday and Wednesday she seemed to make good progress although she was on the critical list until Tuesday. Last Wednesday I was very happy with Rainie's progress.

Thursday [November 12] I was allowed to see her between 7-8pm. I nearly died. She was completely incoherent in deep delirium and had death written all over her face. The Doctor was working with her and said shock had set in and she was fast using the strength she needed so badly. He said, I can't see how she can possibly live. All I can do is pray for guidance. I wouldn't give you 2 cents for her chances."

I had to keep up the front till after I got the children home and in bed, then I went to hell. It was like that Thursday, Friday, and Saturday. Sunday, I felt that I had been able to penetrate the fog a little and drive home the point that she had to *rest, rest, rest*. Sedatives had done no good and it had to be imbedded in her mind that she *had* to rest.

Monday was a little less restless. Tuesday about the same but last night she did get a little sleep. Today [Wednesday, November 18] she was almost completely rational and seemed somewhat relaxed. I spent nearly two hours with

79

her and she talked a little. Most of the time was spent in my assuring her that she had been very sick and all the things she had talked about were a terrible nightmare and she must erase them from her mind and relax and rest and build up strength. Tonight I feel somewhat encouraged.

Much later, Rainie looked back on the whole experience with her usual sardonic sense of humor.

Tongue in Cheek
By
Rainie Clarke

Aside from "cancer", "bubonic plague", and "past-due — please remit", I suppose 'observation polio' is the most dreaded phrase in the English language. The ultimate diagnosis of "Anterior Poliomylitis" is the crack of doom and a life sentence rolled into one. The problems it creates combine the elements of perpetual motion and chain-reaction. One problem leads to another. They are never-ending and they reach out and affect not only the members of one's immediate family, but friends, neighbors and unsuspecting strangers as well.

In my case, the first strangers to be affected were two ambulance attendants. They arrived one Sunday noon, All Saints Day to be precise, having been summoned by a doctor who strongly suspected that I might have polio. Considering the fact that I had already lost the use of my left leg and back muscles, this was not exactly speculation on his part, though there were other possibilities. At any rate, he determined to send me to the county hospital for observation.

On their arrival, the attendants clumped up the narrow stairwell of our house. This stairwell is a relic of the "Roaring '20s" and was designed in the spirit of the flapper figure. Anyone weighing more than 150 pounds must take a deep breath and hold it for

45 seconds in order to get up or downstairs. Too hasty a descent of the stairs is liable to result in a severe case of the "bends".

The two men walked into the bedroom and surveyed the 200 pound bit of feminine fluff they had been called to remove. One of them began to unfold a portable canvas stretcher while the other sized up situation and patient in the manner of Digger O'Dell.

With the professional dexterity of dockwallopers loading sides of beef, my ministering angels dumped my limp and leaden body on the stretcher. They picked it up with a grunt and marched down the railroad hall to the head of the stairs. At this point we made a grim discovery. There was no room in which to turn the stretcher at right angles to the hall to make the descent. Even if this maneuver were possible, the incline was so steep as to expose the first man to an avalanche of quivering femininity. So we all backtracked like a freight train on a siding.

My husband and my two navigators regrouped for action. They rejected the idea of lowering me out of a window like a baby grand piano on the grounds that it was impractical (and who knows, maybe not medically ethical?). They finally tied me into a straight chair and carried me down, practically pick-a-back.

My three children stood by the front door, looking like an illustration for Oliver Twist. I hazily remember bidding them a moist farewell and warning them to brush their teeth and mind Daddy, as the two attendants prepared to load their cargo.

They transferred me to the stretcher and we single-filed out of the house, down the steps, across the lawn, and out to the ambulance. The attendants lifted the litter and shoved it into place, uncomfortably like a slab in the morgue. I was off on the first leg of an adventure that was to last better than a year and a half.

After the confusion of banging doors, elevators, long tile corridors, bustling starched uniforms, and a babble of voices had subsided, I came to the realization that I was lying on a hospital bed. Before I had time to orient myself, a fresh group of voices advanced to the side of my bed, and there remains with me the vague recollection of the cherubic face of an oriental doctor who observed the social amenities by assuring me that "This won't hurt velly much". While two starched uniforms held me on my side in a fetal position, he jabbed a needle into my exposed spine.

Although I did not know it then, this procedure is called a spinal tap. Often it must be repeated three or four times before a satisfactory or conclusive diagnosis can be made.

The mob dematerialized, only to give way to a second crew which arrived with an astonishing collection of hospital paraphernalia: bed pans, enema cans, and miles and miles of rubber hose. At this point I lapsed into a merciful oblivion.

Sometime during the middle of the night I became conscious long enough to discover that the obstruction in my nose was a nasal catheter leading to an oxygen tank.

At eight o'clock the next morning, my room became an ant hill of activity. Uniforms rustled, voices percolated, and it seemed to me that even my bed had joined in the general merriment and was rolling facetiously out into the hall. This was not a product of my imagination. The Uniforms had taken hold of both ends of my bed and were propelling it and me down the long corridor with a rapidity faintly reminiscent of my usually hectic trips to the delivery room.

No matter what elaborate plans I may have made to avoid such circumstances, most of my life Fate has intervened to create last-minute havoc. In three journeys to the delivery table, not one of them was made in a calm and orderly manner. I have finally resigned myself to this state of affairs, and I don't even try to do my Christmas shopping early anymore.

We arrived in a large room at the end of the hall amidst much excitement. The nurses and attendants parked my bed next to an open respirator. After much exertion, they managed to roll me uphill onto the respirator mattress. They told me later that, due to my obesity, the whole performance took on an atmosphere of stuffing sausage into a casing. Had I weighed another five pounds, all bets would have been off. To their everlasting credit, they did get me bolted into that iron corset, and the weirdest episode of my life was under way.

Ordinarily you do not enter an iron lung until all other methods have failed and you are doing a credible job of imitating a blue-point oyster. Once you are inside the hull, it is obvious to you that no bi-valve was ever more securely encased.

The next item in the long list of things being done to and for me, was the administering of an IV (intravenous feeding). The glucose and saline solution was placed in its rack and the needle inserted in the vein on the inside of my right elbow. This was then taped in place and my arm was pinioned to the bed to prevent my disturbing the flow. As it turned out, this was an unnecessary precaution. I couldn't have moved my right arm under any circumstances. I had lost all motion in it.

I had been warned that the IV would take approximately eight hours. Now, I can think of a great many ways by which eight hours can be stretched into infinity, including a Sunday afternoon visit from your in-laws; but few of them can compare with lying on your back, with your throat in a vise, waiting for a half-gallon of fluid to enter your system drop by drop.

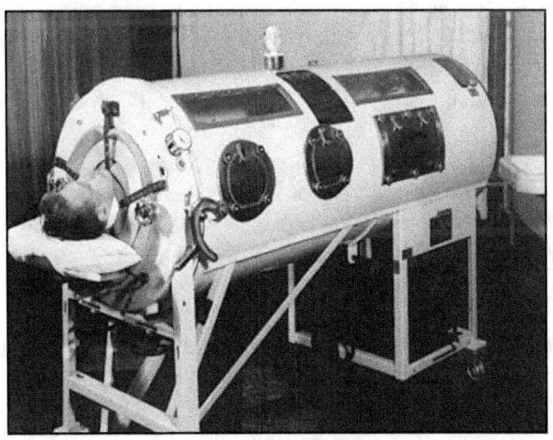

Despite even these frightful recollections, no one who hasn't "been there" can visualize the loneliness, fear, and ostracism those quarantined because of polio faced at the time. Neighbors shunned the family; the mailman, milk delivery man, and others would not even approach the house, but left their packages on the curb of the street. Brave and generous souls would sometime leave a bag of food on the porch, ring the doorbell, then quickly escape before anyone could come to the door. The Clarkes' Thanksgiving dinner in 1953 was delivered in exactly that manner.

A quarantine sign. The original was bright red-orange.

The children were not able to see their mother between the time she left for the hospital on November 1, 1953 until the beginning of March, 1954, more than four months. Even then, they were allowed only five to fifteen minute visits once a week. When he finally got to visit his mother, Timmy, then still under three years old, was terribly worried because "Mommy hasn't any shoes on— her foots get cold," according to a letter written by John to thank the children of two junior high school classes that had donated presents for the children's Christmas. Those presents included a pair of slippers for Rainie and at a subsequent visit, John, Chris, and Timmy made sure to put the slippers on Rainie's feet.

Even long after the quarantine had been lifted, people were wary of interaction with family members, afraid to shake hands or stop by for a visit. As much as a year later, as Toby's 8th birthday

84

came around, John had to send a letter to the parents of the children he invited to her party:

Dear Mother and Daddy,

I feel it my duty to acquaint you with the following facts in connection with Toby's Invitation to your little daughter.

You're no doubt aware that Rainie, Toby's Mommy, is in Bergen Pines with polio — was stricken last Nov. 1st. June 27, in honor of our Chris' 5th birthday she was home just long enough for dinner. Toby's birthday, October 16, precedes our 13th Anniversary by two days. Consequently it will be an important week-end at our house. And our greatest present is the Doctors allowing Mommy her first week-end home in a year. The ambulance will bring her Saturday morning and return her Sunday afternoon. I'm making the sun porch into her room so that she can be part of the party — Toby's first.

There is absolutely NO DANGER in the contact between our Mommy and your daughter. The ONLY DANGER EVER is during the incubation period or the first couple of weeks after being stricken. Naturally IF there was any danger whatever we would certainly not expose our own three children, much less yours or any other. However, Rainie and I felt we should write you this note so there would be no confusion if your youngster came home from the party and mentioned the word POLIO. We're looking forward to seeing your daughter along with the rest of Toby's class.

Sincerely,

Johnny Clarke

P.S. Incidentally dungarees or slacks are advisable since 5 or 6 RHS [Ridgewood High School] Seniors are going to take the youngsters for a "Nature Hike" in our woods, winding up in the back yard roasting wieners and marshmallows — or if rain, In the basement.

The Long Road Home

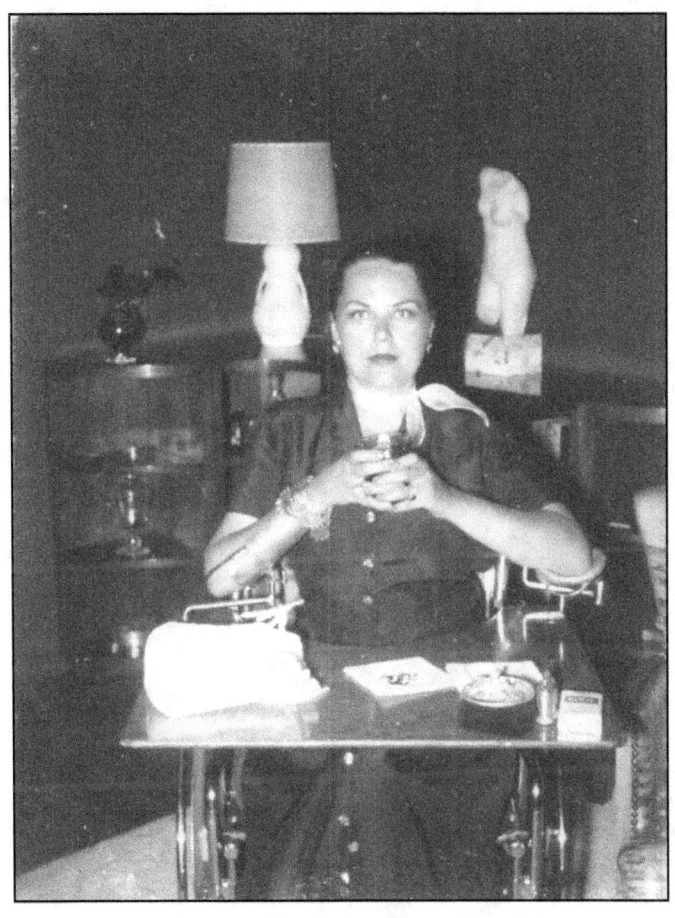

Previous page: Rainie at Warm Springs, 1956, showing her slimmed down look and confidence after almost six months of rehabilitation in the best polio facility in the world.

And thus began Rainie's long struggle—first to emerge from the Iron Lung, then to breathe on her own, to regain some measure of functionality, and finally to return home. The process was to take more than a year-and-a-half.

Rainie left little by way of description of her time in Bergen Pines. She spent five months in the iron lung, one of six in the facility, including both Thanksgiving and Christmas of 1953. In the ward at the same time were mostly younger patients, some of whom spent the remainder of their lives in these artificial respirators. Altogether, according to press reports, she was one of 140 cases of polio in Bergen County, New Jersey in 1953, the highest total for any New Jersey county.

Smoke and mirrors

In addition to taking care of the three children and trying to put the new house in order, John continued to work in radio and commercial recording as jobs were available. He spent as much time as possible visiting with Rainie. The stubbornness that helped get her through her ordeal was also manifest in a less desirable manner. Long before the days of "no smoking" buildings, smoking cigarettes in public spaces—even hospitals—was common, as shown in Rainie's description of John's agonizing wait for word of his wife's fate. But smoking around lung-impaired patients or those on supplemental oxygen was *verboten*. Nonetheless, Rainie, a lifelong smoker, with the connivance of her husband, managed to continue to "enjoy" her habit even while in the iron lung. John would sneak in cigarettes and a lighter, hold the cigarette for Rainie to inhale, and hide the ashes and butts in a small, plastic cosmetic case which he would take with him when he left. Rainie stopped smoking, though it is unclear whether at Bergen Pines or after arriving at Warm Springs, but in March 1955 back-slid and resumed, a habit she continued until her death.

Locked tightly in the neck-embrace of the respirator, the only way the patient could see anything or communicate with visitors was by means of mirrors arranged above her head or sometimes on the side of the iron lung. In this way, for five months, Rainie's life truly became a metaphor for the ephemeral human existence, one of smoke and mirrors.

On the home front

       John had only intermittent, part time work and faced the unpalatable tradeoff between paying the high cost of a professional adult babysitter while he worked late evenings and nights at WOR in New York City or taking off work and forgoing the income. The family's financial plight was truly precarious, partially alleviated only by the charity and kindness of friends, neighbors, the West Side Presbyterian Church, the Junior Women's Club of Ridgewood, and a few other local organizations. Sad to say, John later told his children, the local chapter of the Red Cross was not one of those who sprang to help. He maintained that the only assistance the local chapter—as opposed to the National Red Cross—had ever provided was "one chipped enamel bedpan" after Rainie returned home.

       Among the stalwarts of support were Mrs. John J. ("Betty") Newberry, Jr., Chairwoman of Ridgewood's 1954 March of Dimes campaign and the wife of the owner of one of the largest department stores in Bergen County. Over the next several years, she and several other kindly and generous folks brought innumerable bags of clothes—often taking them home to alter the sizes to fit the children as they grew—as well as food, toys, and Christmas presents for the children. Dr. Arthur M. Hughes, pastor of the West Side Presbyterian Church, also provided spiritual and practical counseling and coordinated financial and other assistance to the struggling Clarkes.

      Among the more remarkable volunteers was a group of teenaged girls from the YWCA's service group who spent untold hours providing free babysitting so John could visit Rainie, go shopping, or go to work. On June 3, 1954, the *Ridgewood Herald-News* ran a front page article about these selfless young ladies:

Y-Girls 'Mother' Tots
Whose Mom Has Polio

Anyone who has let all the talk about juvenile delinquency convince him that the country's young people are all going to the dogs should talk to John H. Clarke of 177 [sic., 174] Mountain Avenue, Ridgewood.

Three Children

For several months, now, teen-age girls from the Ridgewood YWCA's service group have been operating a free baby-sitting service for Mr. Clarke, who has three small children. His 33-year-old wife, Rainie, has been in Bergen Pines Hospital since last November 1, with polio.

The future looked pretty bleak for Mr. Clarke, left at home with three small children in a community where he knew almost no one.

His work complicated things even further, because he is an announcer-narrator at WOR Channel 9 in New York, and works nights.

He was struggling with the problem of hiring baby-sitters every night, and Sundays, so he could visit his wife, when some teenagers at the Y heard of his plight and volunteered to help.

Nancy Drier is chairman of the service group that has been proving to anyone who is interested that not all juveniles think only in terms of themselves.

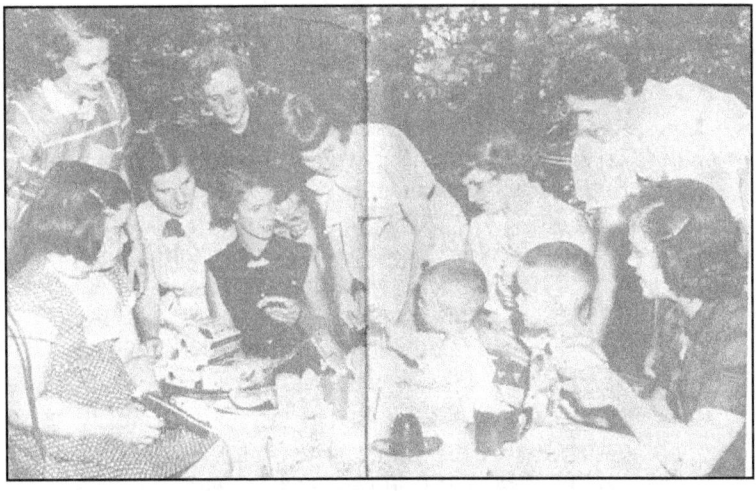

Clarke family birthday party, June 1954. (Clockwise) Toby Clarke, Ann Jones, Ann Brockheusen, Ann Colgan, Jane Hopken, Nancy Drier, Jane Annan, Karen Olson, Dottie Floyd. (At the table) Tim and Chris Clarke. (Ridgewood Herald News, June 3, 1954.)

<u>Work Regularly</u>

Nancy said about 75 Ridgewood area girls have helped with the baby-sitting. They come to the Clarke home regularly on Sundays, and Mr. Clarke says they are more faithful than many grown women who keep house for money.

Although Mr. Clarke hires other baby-sitters during the week, the girls from the Y also come over frequently at other times to help out.

"They make a party out of it," said the grateful father, as he explained how they pack a picnic lunch, dress the children, pile into the family car and amuse the children on the hospital grounds while Mr. Clarke visits with his wife in the building. Children are not permitted in the building but there are times when Mrs. Clarke can wave to them from the porch window.

The Clarke children look upon the girls as older sisters, and obviously enjoy all the attention they get.

The youngsters are Toby, 7, whose real name is October; Chris, 5, and Timmy, who was the happy guest of honor at a birthday party arranged Tuesday afternoon by some dozen of the attractive young Samaritans.

Toby was named October because she was born on October 16, two days before the Clarkes' anniversary on October 18.

Despite the generosity of many in the community, the Clarkes' finances were in desperate straits. As John wrote in a September 22, 1954 letter to the head of the Bergen County chapter of the National Foundation for Infantile Paralysis,

> Only part-time work [has been] available through the winter and I looked forward to a good increase in the summer. The past three summers I had worked 26 weeks each summer for Mutual [WOR]. This summer an efficiency expert did away with mine and six other jobs. Added expense of baby sitters and other necessary items have more than used all available monies. Neither of us have families to help and although I'm very happy to do all the washing, ironing, cooking, etc., myself, it does become necessary to take the youngsters with me or have baby sitters each time I leave the house.

In an early February 1955 letter to Rainie, John let on just how strained the family's resources were:

> Toby was home since it was a short day and school was out at 12:45. Then of course LUNCH. With this MOB only soup will streettcchtt so everybody had two bowls of soup....spaghetti & sauce left from Sat., rice left from Sun. and a can of mixed vegetables -- oh yes, a few BLACK EYED PEAS left from one nite last week.

Rainie improves

As winter turned to spring, and then into summer, Rainie began making slow progress. First, she was allowed out of the iron lung for short periods of a few minutes at a time to re-learn to breathe on her own. After five months, she was transferred to a "rocking bed," a device that uses gravity to assist the diaphragm to contract and relax, making breathing less reliant on purely muscle capacity alone. By the fall of 1954, she apparently was able to go for periods of time without the assistance of the rocking bed, and by the summer of 1955, was even allowed out for short visits home.

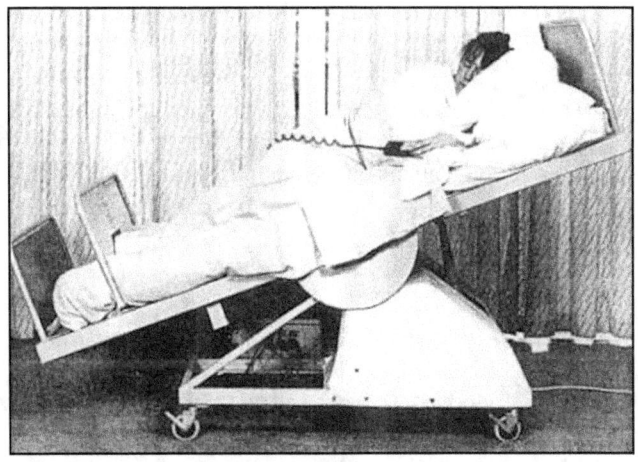

A rocking bed.

Working for the Cause

With their typical energy and optimism, John and Rainie got to work—she on her rehabilitation, he on caring for the family, working when work was available, and both on throwing their support behind the March of Dimes and its Red Feather Drive fund raiser. In January 1954, Mrs. John J. Newberry, Jr., Chairwoman of Ridgewood's 1954 March of Dimes campaign, asked John to write a letter "to add his pleas to the campaign," according to an article in the January 10 edition of the *Ridgewood Sunday News*. John's letter was heartfelt and eloquent:

January 6, 1954

Letters to the Editor
Ridgewood Sunday News
Ridgewood, New Jersey

Dear Sir:

Chris, my four-and-a-half [year-old], says, " I just hate that old word POLIO. Every time I hear it I get fightin' mad." The poor little guy has good reason to feel that way too. It has been 10 weeks today (Sunday) since he's seen his mommy. Oh no, Chris, thank God, is hale and hearty — his MOMMY has polio.

I sincerely hope you, reader, shall never find it necessary to call your little brood together to tell them "Mommy has polio!" Can you imagine what it means to tell a family that? Let your imagination run rampant for a minute. Now, triple your most nightmarish conclusions and you're nearly right.

Hospitals were old stuff to me. I thought I was pretty blasé about illnesses. Well, maybe not blasé, but I had been around and thought I could take it in my stride. I've had the pleasure of playing every hospital within 75 miles of New York in the last 10 years. You see a lot of illness that way, you know. I even imagined I knew a good bit about polio –

I ' d played many Saturday afternoon shows at Warm Springs where I'd seen it in every stage. But, I hadn't *lived with it*.

And you know a very odd thing happened when our family started living with polio. I learned the value of a DIME. Have you ever stopped to think what a dime can buy? No — not for you — for a polio patient?? — a respirator (maybe you call it an iron lung); braces; a wheelchair; the salary of a thera-pist, so the braces and chair won't be permanent; a nurse to stand by your side when you can't even breathe for yourself; a swimming pool — or even more important, DIMES pay for RE-SEARCH to find that "ounce of prevention", instead of the costly and painful months of cure.

Above I've said, "our family started living with polio" — that gets to be a pretty big family when polio strikes your home — a family which includes your friends, your church and the NATIONAL FOUNDATION FOR INFANTILE PARALYSIS, as well as your Doc-tors and nurses. Believe me, you'll be glad to have every one of them in your corner. I don't know what we'd have done without the church and National Foundation. After a couple of weeks, when my wife had a turn for the worse, National Foundation, watching her closely, brought in special nurses around the clock to make sure she had every possible chance. They're ever watchful, looking for a way to help the patient or aid the family. Their collective broad shoulder is at the wheel or at your beck and call as a place of refuge and enlightenment . Believe me you'll find you need the help of National Founda-tion — as they need your help now in their 1954 MARCH OF DIMES. GIVE — and hope that it shall NOT BE RETURNED.

Johnny Clarke for
Rainie Clarke (who had her 33rd birthday 11/28 in an iron lung)
Toby Clarke, 7 yr. daughter
Chris Clarke, 4-1/2 yr. son
Timmy Clarke, 2-1/2 yr. son
"Rags and Tatters" (a pair of cocker puppies, who miss her too)

While in the iron lung, Rainie recorded a one-minute radio announcement for the March of Dimes which was later said to have been the campaign's most successful fund-raiser ever. It read:

> My name is Rainie Clarke. On November 1, 1953 I got polio. That same day I learned that the March of Dimes meant *life* to me. Life, and the hope of recovery. When I finish speaking to you, I must go back into the iron lung. Know what I'll be thinking about then? The day when there may be no more infantile paralysis...if this year's March of Dimes is big enough to pay for the mass testing of a new vaccine. You see, I'm a mother of three children, and I know what polio means! That's why I ask you to give to help others in iron lungs...then give again so there need *be* no more iron lungs. Please join the 1954 March of Dimes!

John and Rainie used all their talents to raise awareness and funds for the anti-polio campaign. Over the summer and fall, they worked on a one-act play to be presented at the October 1954 rally to start the following year's March of Dimes campaign. (See pages 99-103.) Again, their efforts were recognized in a front-page article in the *Ridgewood Herald-News* (October 7, 1954):

Polio Victim Pens Red Feather Skit

They'll laugh when the Midland Park—Ho-Ho-Kus—Ridgewood Community Chest puts on the skit, "Hired, Tired Feather," at the annual Kickoff Rally on October 13.

The skit is one of 12 big acts to be put on at the Ridgewood High School auditorium to launch the record-breaking Red Feather drive which goes into full operation the middle of the month.
The chances are that Johnny Clarke would laugh, too, with the rest of the capacity audience which is expected to be on hand. So would his daughter, Toby, 8, and his two "All-boy" sons—Chris, 5, and Timmy, 3.
But they probably won't be there.

Won't Be There

Rainie Clarke would laugh too (and this may not sound modest because she wrote the skit). But it's for sure she won't be there.

Let's go back...

A year ago, Rainie, Johnny, Toby, Chris, and Timmy moved from a small apartment in New York to the home of their dreams at 174 Mountain Avenue in Ridgewood.

"Nothing fancy as you can see," says Johnny, "but just what Rainie wanted for the children."

That was September 1, 1953.

Less than a month later [sic., actually two months], Rainie was stricken with polio.

Today, she is still in Bergen Pines Hospital. And the plain truth of the matter is that Rainie still has a long way to go. Rainie can move her left arm because she has fought the good fight. She can move only the fingers of her right hand.

This writing game, as anyone can tell you, is a tough game. Comedy is even tougher, even if you have facility in both hands and a couple of heads.

The Hard Way

Rainie did it the hard way. With a little strength in her left hand, she grasped a long-handled salad mixing spoon and thrust it across her stomach to her right hand. She has no strength in her right arm yet, but with the fingers she can move on her right hand, she can grasp the spoon. Then, with her left hand she pulls the right hand over to a writing position. The good nurses put a sandbag under the right elbow to keep the arm up and Rainie begins writing.

She can't move the right arm so she prints one letter and then pulls the writing pad one space to the left so to speak.

That's the way the skit, "Hired, Tired Feather," was written. It tells the story of a Community Chest solicitor and the comic troubles he had with one of his calls. All fictions, of course.

When it was all printed, Johnny typed it up.

"You may wonder why we would do this," Johnny said. "It's this. This was our first real home. (The way he said it made you want to live here forever.) We can't contribute much monetarily to the Chest. As you can see, I've quite a family to take care of."

That's why Rainie, Johnny, Toby, Chris and Timmy won't be

there. Neither will "Rags" and "Tatters", their two dogs, one of whom chews up nearly everything in the house, and we're not going to put the finger on which one.

Because he's the "housekeeper" as well as the "breadwinner", even the problem of going downtown for a package of cigarettes is a major operation for Johnny Clarke, what with rounding up the kids and getting the dogs in the cellar.

But the Clarkes are not easily discouraged. Their big hope now—and they are both veterans of the radio and television field—is to launch a really adult man-wife program of their own, possibly via home-to-hospital telephone, to give hope to others who also have serious problems.

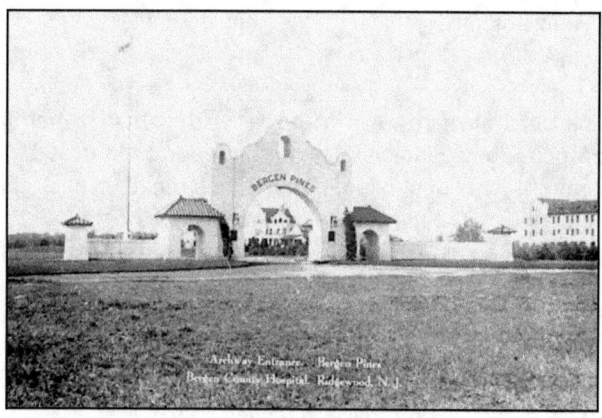

Entrance to Bergen Pines Hospital, 1950s.

"A HIRED, TIRED FEATHER"
A ONE ACT PITCH
IN ONE SCENE
Rainie Clarke

SCENE: Living room of the Van Ridgely home.
TIME: Optional

SCENE OPENS on a living room furnished in traditional style. Main props are desk and telephone, CENTER-FRONT. Desk is covered with an assortment of papers. OFFSTAGE, RIGHT, a radio is blaring the latest nonsensical version of a literary genius type lyric entitled, "Sh-- Boom". As the CURTAIN RISES, MRS. WOODROW VAN RIDGELY is standing at the desk, phone in hand. The vacuum cleaner is lying idle in the middle of the floor, STAGERIGHT. As the scene progresses, events approach near pandemonium!

(THE CURTAIN RISES)

Mrs. WVR: (She is dressed neatly with apron and dust cap for protection).

"Hello - Acme employment? This is Mrs. Woodrow Van Ridgely. Have you someone you can send me to do a little *light* house cleaning? Oh, dear, I've been so busy with committee meetings and school starting — and — well, you know how it is — and — well, tonight I'm having an executive committee meeting for the Red Feather drive — and my fall housecleaning isn't finished, and — Oh! A MAN? ... Oh well, I suppose, if it's ALL you've got — yes, right away — 1954 Van Gogh Blvd."

(She replaces the phone, picks up vacuum cleaner, and starts on the walls. DOOR BELL RINGS. She puts down vacuum, leaving it running - and starts to answer the door -- gets halfway between CENTERSTAGE and DOOR, STAGE LEFT, when PHONE RINGS --- she calls to door:) "Just a minute, please" — as she returns to desk and PICKS up PHONE.

Mrs. WVR: "Hello. Yes---yes, I called - it's about the television set. I want someone to come over right away — but — but — but, my dear man — do you realize I've had to resort to listening to the

99

RADIO? (She speaks the last word as if it had an unpleasant taste.) — Right away? (She beams) Oh fine!"

(She REPLACES PHONE and MOVES to DOOR. OPENS DOOR to find standing on the threshold a nice looking, mild mannered, very tired gentleman, with *very tired feet* — and what appears to be an armful of canvassing equipment. He might even be called a Stan Laurel type. Mrs. Van R. motions him inside as she dives to answer the phone again. During her ensuing conversation tired man MOVES into room, DOWNSTAGE LEFT of desk, unnoticed by Mrs. Van R.)

Mrs. WVR: "Hello? Oh, hello, Agnes! My dear, I'm simply up to my ears! Well, you know how it is when you're on so many committees. You did the same thing last year, yourself – Yes, I'm having the committee here tonight – and Woodrow's having a fit. You know what he says about committees: a bunch of people who keep minutes and waste hours! Agnes, listen, do you know if Irene is coming? Well, if there's one thing to be said for free advice, it's worth it! Just a minute, Agnes, I smell something burning. (She turns to Tired Man and says;)

"Run out to the kitchen and see what's burning!" (She beckons him with her forefinger - then during the following business she tries to juggle the phone between her ear and shoulder while she continues to talk.)

"You know, Agnes, I really feel that the drive this year — (She's busy removing her apron and dropping it over Tired Man's head.) — is as important as it has ever been! Don't you? And I really feel that the only way to *do* things — (here she punctuates each word with tying the apron bow - ending the tying and sentence simultaneously) -- **is - to - get - things - done**!

(With pat on the back she partially shoves Tired Man toward kitchen door.) "Yes — yes, I know that's the trouble with Irene — well you know I wouldn't say anything about her unless I could say something good -- and, oh *brother* -- is this good!"

(Just then Tired Man comes in from kitchen with large
wooden cooking spoon, as if to ask directions — and
DOORBELL RINGS. Meanwhile radio has long since
changed to other tunes.)

Tired Man: "Please Ma'am…"

Mrs. WVR: (To Tired Man) "Would you please see who's at the
door?"

(Back to phone.) "Now where was I? (Tired Man crosses
to front door STAGELEFT. Opens door to admit TV repairman).

TV man: "Ok, where's the set?" (He steps inside, carrying his tool
kit.)

Mrs. WRV: "OH, (To repairman) it's right over here." (She points
to set DOWNSTAGE RIGHT)

"Well, as I was about to tell you, Agnes — (Tired Man has
come DOWNSTAGE LEFT to his equipment again, and is
sorting through cards) — "Irene was telling Fred about her
experiences collecting for last year's drive, and she says to
Fred: 'Fred, if that woman yawned once she yawned a
dozen times,' and do you know what Fred said? He said,
'Maybe she wasn't yawning, Irene. Maybe she was trying
to say something!' Isn't that rich? Irene talks more than
any woman I know."

(BACK door buzzer BUZZES. Mrs. WVR to Tired Man
who has been standing at her elbow with spoon tucked
under his arm and cards in one hand vainly trying to get
her attention) — "That's the back door. Will you see who
it is, please?"

(Tired Man reluctantly goes out kitchen door.)

"I know it: Just yesterday I asked her if she had mentioned
to Fred what you told me.....and she said...."...Why, darling, no. *I didn't tell anyone — I didn't know it was a secret!*"

101

(Tired Man reenters from the kitchen and comes down toward desk closely followed by the plumber.)

Tired Man: "Mrs. Van Ridgely – uh, pardon me. Mrs. Van Ridgley, it's the plumber…"

Mrs. WVR: "Oh, yes -- take him out to the kitchen and show him the sink. It seems to be clogged."

(Tired Man and the plumber exit to kitchen.) (Mrs. WVR gets back to Agnes:)

"Well, Agnes - Irene is simply a riot! We were discussing prices and budgets and Irene was bemoaning the fact that she can never stay within hers - and she looked at me with a perfectly straight face and said , 'I really don't want a lot of money, but I wish we could afford to live the way we're living now!' (She laughs as the FRONT DOOR BELL RINGS, immediately followed by a loud BANGING on the kitchen pipes, indicating that the plumber is testing the reflexes of the kitchen plumbing.)

Mrs. WVR: "Hold on a minute, Agnes, I have to answer the front door. My cleaning man is in the kitchen with the plumber." (She puts down the phone and crosses to front door. She admits a nice pleasant man in overalls. Precisely as Mrs. WVR opens the door Tired Man marches in from the kitchen with a determined look in his eye.)

Cleaner: "How d'ydo? Madam, I'm the man front the Acme Employment Company."
Mrs. WVR: "Oh! But you can't be! You're out in the kitchen!" (Tired Man has crossed to just right of CENTER STAGE. Mrs. WVR turns to head for the kitchen and sees him. She has reached CENTER STAGE with the cleaner right behind.)

"Well, then, for goodness sakes, who are YOU?"

Tired Man: "I'm the canvasser for the RED FEATHER DRIVE."

Mrs. WVR: (She sits at the desk, picks up a pen, and

makes out a check. During all of this Tired Man is
removing the apron and collecting his stuff to leave).

Mrs. WVR: "Well, my dear man, you mustn't hide *that* light under
a bushel! You know it's vitally important for you to get
your message across — After all, nobody is going to refuse
if you let them know you're from the RED FEATHER!
(She finishes check and hands it to him with a flourish. He
accepts it gratefully and makes his exit as hastily as possible.)

Mrs. WVR: (To cleaner, on resumption of banging on kitchen
pipes:) "You might as well take the cleaner — (she
indicates) — and finish the walls." (He starts to work as
she picks up the phone.)

"Hello, Agnes, you still there? — Honestly, Agnes, I've
finally come to the conclusion that if you want — (here
she is beckoning the cleaner and repeating the business of
putting the apron on him, while juggling the telephone) —
"a thing done right you *simply have to do it yourself*!"

(FAST CURTAIN)

Taking the Next Step—Off to Warm Springs

While Rainie was struggling to improve and regain the
ability to breathe unassisted, John was quietly working behind the
scenes to try to arrange for her to be admitted to the famous Warm
Springs Foundation in Warm Springs, Georgia. Founded by the late
President Franklin D. Roosevelt, who had contracted polio in 1921
at the age of 39, Warm Springs was located on the site of an old
Indian mineral spring that had long been believed to have healing
properties. Roosevelt had bought the run-down vacation resort and
several thousand acres of adjacent property which had long attracted
Atlanta's wealthy, and had converted it into a rehabilitation facility
specifically for polio patients. It was considered the premier polio
rehabilitation facility in the country, but was extremely difficult to
get into given the high demand, not only within the U.S. but around
the world.

Working quietly though Warm Springs' director of admissions, Fred Botts; the National Foundation for Infantile Paralysis (both the Bergen County chapter and the national headquarters); Rainie's doctors at Bergen Pines; and pulling every string he could think of among his contacts in the entertainment community; by late 1954 John had arranged for Rainie to be admitted as an in-patient for rehabilitation. Rainie, however, had to be free of the need for any assisted breathing, including the rocking bed, for at least 30 days before she was considered qualified. Awaiting that milestone, and then delayed because of acute rooming problems and heavy commitments for bed space at the Foundation, however, Rainie was not to make the trip until the end of the year.

Rainie's admission was something of a sensitive issue due to the family's inability to afford virtually any aspect of the program. John described the family "finances" to a representative from Social Services. In a letter to Rainie, he later explained, enjoining her to keep the information strictly confidential:

> When I told her income, as weighed against absolutely necessary outlay (like babysitter fees, house etc — not even mentioning food, utilities and such) she said, "Why, you can't do that", just house and babysitter from your income only leaves you about $30-40 a month for food. And when you told me at the Dec. 17 call (about the County Chapter) that you only had $25 in the house I was terribly upset. You can't get by with that kind of math. My reply was of course that we were "getting by" and that you can't just sit down and quit because the jig-saw doesn't make a picture this time — it might IF you keep trying. I told her what happened HERE wasn't important, it was what happened to you...
>
> Then out of a clear sky she said, "We don't want either you or Rainie worrying about things, especially ABOUT Rainie. Now this is something which I must tell you in the strictest confidence, and we ask you to tell no one any more about it. It's a wonderful thing and you should be very proud — there is a fund and arrangement whereby Warm Springs can accept a MAXIMUM OF TWO people each year as THEIR GUESTS. In view of all circumstances

Rainie has been chosen to be one of those people.
Beyond her physical condition, Rainie and you have made quite an impression on Warm Springs with your resourcefulness and attitude and we are happy that it could be arranged. We'd like for you to feel that her care and rehabilitation for awhile at least, would not be a worry. We don't know how long it will be necessary for her to be in WS [Warm Springs] but we would want to get her to the point where she can come home from there bypassing any local institution [i.e., directly home, not to a nursing or rehabilitation facility] — but come home to a reasonably normal living.

Rainie arrived at Warm Springs in mid-November, 1954 and John spent a very hurried two days helping her get settled in and meeting with the administration.[1] She spent her 34th birthday there, receiving a telegram from the family. Written correspondence apparently was very limited over the next month-and-a-half, because John and Rainie exchanged Christmas telegrams shortly after the holiday. At that time, long-distance telephone calls were quite expensive, especially on such a strained budget as the Clarkes were facing; it is not clear if there was a Christmas phone call as well.

Rainie and John began to exchange letters by at least January 1, 1955, with Rainie laboriously writing hers out long hand. John retyped much of her correspondence and circulated it to friends and family between January and March. A number of John's letters to Rainie also survive, unfortunately many of them undated, making it difficult to determine an exact chronology. Their respective letters give a good idea of what each was doing and how each felt during this period.

---

[1] I have not been able to ascertain the exact date she arrived, but it apparently was around November 15. John's hurried visit seems to have been between November 16-18, because by November 19 he was back at work in New York and wrote a letter to an friend in Georgia apologizing for not having met while he was in the state.

Life at Warm Springs

Rainie's letters give a very good idea of the exhaustion of rehabilitation and the exhilaration and joyfulness of living at the Warm Springs Foundation. In late January, for example, she wrote:

Since starting on a functional training program I seem to be on the go all the time. I start with a treatment in the pool at 8:30. Then Martha (my PT - physical therapist) lets me sit in a chair In the pool and stretch myself while she treats some of her of her other patients — so usually I don't get out of the pool till around 10:30. — and by the time I get dressed and back over to the room it's almost 11:00 — and by the time I'm settled comfortably in bed and ready to get some work done the dinner trays arrive.

Right after dinner I have to get my corset on and then turn over for rest hour (about 25 mins. for me). Then the push-boy arrives to take me to mat activities (which is stretching period) at Roosevelt Hall. I have to be there 1:00.

I get back from there (where I'm trying to learn to roll over as well as have my hips stretched — *very* painful, since they hadn't been stretched in 14 months) around two o'clock. They Increased my time up this week to five hours plus meals, so I usually stay up in my chair as I have to go back to Roosevelt Hall for a functional training class at 4:30. This is where they try to teach you to do things for yourself. Right now I'm in a dressing class, trying to learn to put on and take off my corset. I can unfasten and unlace it — also fasten and lace it up — but rolling on and off it and getting it in place is a different problem.

Yesterday I did my own hair for the first time! And all the PTs in class said I did a remarkable job. Last week on my functional test I managed to scoot my left hip forward and get a sliding board under it. My PT was floored! She said she would have bet anything that it was something I would never be able to do. Yesterday she also paid me a compliment of telling the head of functional training that I was amazing as I did almost EVERYTHING with SHEER DETERMINATION as I CERTAINLY DIDN'T have the MUSCLES to do them with! I was highly flattered.

Incidentally, the list of muscles I DON'T HAVE is fairly staggering! I borrowed my PT's "Gray's Anatomy" (it only weighs 8 lbs.) so I could study the muscle, nerve and bone structure to give me a better idea of what I'm doing. For a girl with: NO right arm, NO shoulders, only ONE side, practically NO abdominals, NO hips, NO glutes (fanny, that is) and NO legs, I seem to be doing alright!

After I get back from functional training it's after 5. Supper arrives about 5:15 so I usually stay up until the orderly gets back from his supper hour, sometime around 6:30. Then he puts me back to bed. Sometimes we get up again around 7 or 7:30 and stay up till nine (last nite we all sat out on the sun porch and had a community sing until 9:30) then we are put back to bed and readied tor the night.

Other nights the mob comes to this room — Sunday, 7 wheel chairs. And of course on Monday and Thursday nites are movie nites — I'm looking forward to them more now that I can go in a chair instead of a stretcher. Also I've been attending church services, and yesterday Ruth Nimey took me on a tour of the kitchen over at Georgia Hall where she is supervisor.

I Just finished eating dinner and I have a minute or two left before I have to turn over. Next week I get another new PT as the one I have now has to give up her patients in order to teach students and I understand that I'm to have an extra stretching period added to my schedule.[2]

Among other newsworthy notes — my braces are ready and as soon as my shoes arrive from Columbus I under-

---

[2] In addition to being a major rehabilitation facility, Warm Springs was also a major training facility for physical and occupational therapists and other specialists. There was a steady stream of OT and PT classes passing in and out.

stand they will begin standing me! Also, Just came back from dressing class where, with the aid of an aluminum cane, I pulled myself over in bed and got my slacks all the way off UNASSISTED!! was really proud of that accomplishment!!! Of course it was painstakingly slow — but so is everything else!

Rainie also shared some information about the social and recreational life of Warm Springs, an integral part of the rehabilitative process and one of the unique elements that made the foundation feel like "home" to so many of the patients, some of whom remember the place fondly 50 or 60 years after spending time there.[3]

[Rainie's roommate] claims that everybody on the Foundation knows Rainie — this is quite an exaggeration, but I have met a lot of people and a lot of them call me by my first name, and incidentally, the cover and cartoon for "WHEELCHAIR REVIEW" were received quite well.[4] (Ed. [John's interjection] Rainie was chosen staff cartoonist for monthly publication). I'm working now on the Feb. issue.

They have an organization here for staff members only,

[3.] The author was able to contact one gentleman, now in his early 70s, who had been a patient at Warm Springs twice as an early teenager in the early 1950s. He fondly remembered such things as the fancy dining room, illicit wheelchair races down the long, sloping sidewalk in the central square, and the sound of the winds blowing through the pines—a sound he said reminded him of the ocean. His only negative memory was—interestingly—a visit by Eleanor Roosevelt, wife of FDR, the founder of the institution. The kids had earned the privilege of watching the World Series on the foundation's *new* black-and-white television, but the staff turned off the game when Mrs. Roosevelt entered. For a 13-year-old, watching the *World Series* and *on TV* was a far bigger deal than meeting the former first lady!

[4.] The "Wheelchair Review" was a mimeographed periodical put out on an irregular basis by patients and staff that contained news of comings and goings, scheduled activities at the Foundation, writings, book reviews, poems, cartoons, jokes, and other contributions by patients, and a children's section. It was published at least from the early to the late 1950s. The staff archivist in 2010 was kind enough to provide the author with electronic copies of remaining issues (an incomplete collection, unfortunately).

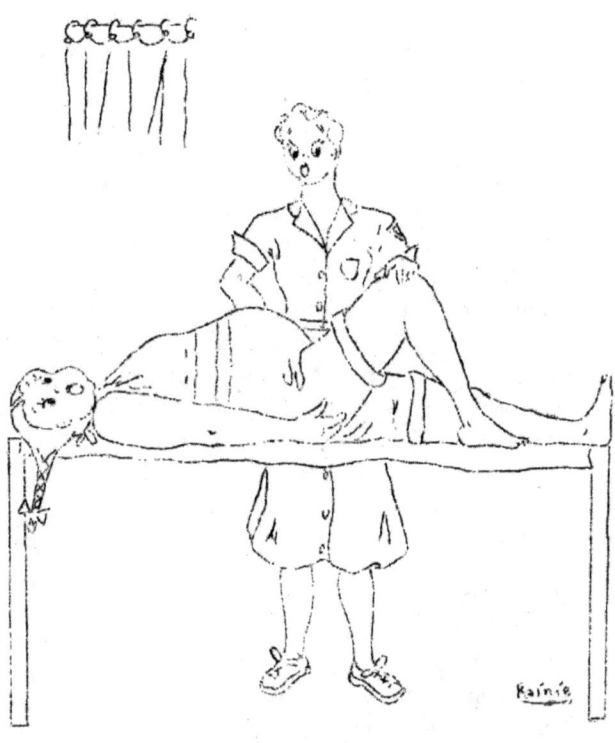

"Pee Tee"

"Believe Me, Miss Murgatroyd, it's Quads!"

One of Rainie's drawings for the "Wheelchair Review," March 12, 1955.

called The Pine Cone Players — but they have asked me if I will give them lessons in make-up — and you know the ham in me! Of course I said yes! So will you please buy a fresh box of nose putty, a brown eyebrow pencil, and put as much stuff in my make-up as possible from the other kits, including crepe hair and spirit gum, then mail me the key and ship the make-up kit as soon as you possibly can? I'm quite excited to be included in this last activity, as it does not ordinarily include the patients.

(In early March) Last Tuesday night I went to the Pine Cone Players auditions and helped them chose their cast for the spring production — a mystery —"The Green Light". And, Wednesday nite was QUITE a nite — my PT (who is an Army Captain, stationed at Valley Forge Hospital) will be leaving the end of the month. She is a photography hobbyist — so she invited me to come up to her cottage after supper to see some of her 35mm color slides. Well, it's the first time I've visited anybody's house but ours (twice) in a year and a half - what a Big Deal!

Rainie's physical progress continued apace. In early March, she wrote:

So many things have happened this week and so many of your unanswered questions keep rolling over in my mind that I hardly know where to begin. This past week has really been quite strenuous and I for one was glad to see Saturday arrive if only to rest up for an equally strenuous one next week. I am on a full functional training program now. Among the more notable things I have been able to accomplish: with the aid of an aluminum cane I can pull myself over in bed (a wide bed that is) also remove my slax [slacks] entirely and unfasten and unlace my corset as well as fasten and lace it; with the same cane, put my foot up on a low bed, get the other foot up on a footstool; take the arm off my [wheel]chair and roll into bed!! I was quite proud of this latter trick — although getting back INTO the chair is quite another thing.

Yesterday they fitted my braces and STOOD ME ON MY FEET for the <u>FIRST TIME IN 15 MONTHS</u> on dry land!! I am definitely two inches taller and the floor looked mighty far away! After a few minor adjustments they [the braces] were ready today and I tried them again this morning (naturally someone had to hold me up). However, I'm planning to send them back to the brace shop as they have one glaring oversight. They forgot to put the "E" on CLARKE. I have more trouble with that E.[5]

As for what the Doctors have to say: it isn't much, as about the only time I see them is once a month at Clinic and I've told you the results of those. I am due to go again about the 1st. The reason Dr. Bennett put me on a FULL functional program was that he felt I wasn't losing weight fast enough to warrant staying on a conservative program. I am under the impression that at this late date they do not expect much further return of muscle power, which is the primary reason for teaching me the best methods of using what I have... I made my weekly trek to the scales this morning to discover, much to my delight, that I had lost 3 lbs. last week (had gained 1 the week before) and now weigh in at 142 ... after dieting arduously all week ... thus obviating the necessity of slitting my throat.

Rainie was at Warm Springs for one of the more memorable occurrences of 1955:

It is now Sunday afternoon rest hour, 12:30 to be precise — and about an hour ago it started to snow, a nice gentle fall, which so far does not show much signs of sticking, though the top of the grass is somewhat powdery. You have never heard such excitement! This is obviously

---

[5.] The brace shop at Warm Springs was world-renowned for the skill and ingenuity with which its technicians—especially the head of the shop, who worked there for more than 50 years—were able to manufacture and adapt a wide variety of braces and other adaptive equipment for the patients. The shop also functioned as a training facility for other prosthetics makers. Rainie was referring to the fact that many people incorrectly spelled her last name "Clark", leaving off the final "e."

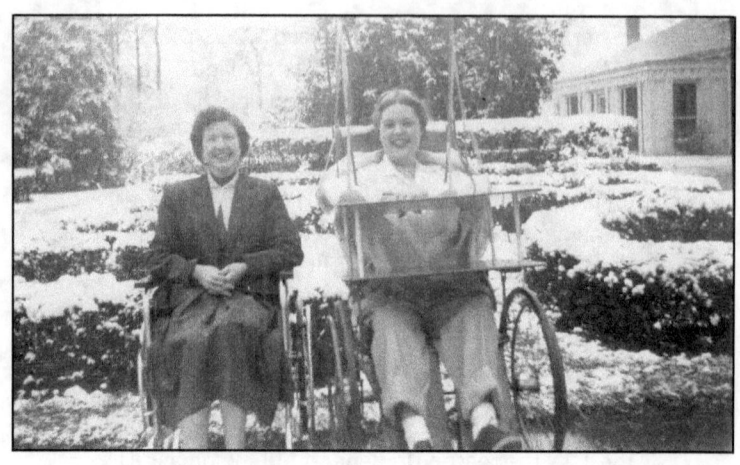

Rainie with a fellow patient during a rare Warm Springs, Georgia
snowstorm, February 1955.

unusual for Warm Springs and I created a light pandemonium by suggesting that it wasn't really SNOW at all, but
rather a midwinter display of cotton blossoms. It looks so
strange to see the green lawn showing thru the powder as
though someone had inadvertently spilled confectioners
sugar...

[Apparently, the area received another snowstorm on
Monday evening-Tuesday morning.] We did get out and
took a few pictures of the storm (which incidentally turned
out to be beautiful — the trees all looked like white lace
and the Campus was a glorious sight — everybody went
wild taking pix and throwing snowballs — it had all melted
this morning).

From Rainie's letters, one can tell that she thoroughly enjoyed the social life at Warm Springs, despite missing her family.
As she related in late January:

Sunday nite they had Fellowship hour over in Georgia Hall.
They had planned to have a song fest, and one of the
Doctors played accompaniment, so Wynelle and I decided

to go. We sat next to the piano and I joined in with my female baritone - whereupon, shortly, Dr. Goslin asked me if I knew "A Good Man Is Hard To Find". The end result was that I sang both that and "Some Of These Days" solo to the crowd — and my reception was in the line of a small ovation - If I do have to say it MYSELF - what a HAM I am! I thoroughly enjoyed every minute of it. Apparently Dr. Goslin did also — as later he suggested that we should get together some time soon and rehearse some numbers.

Along with her active social life, Rainie continued the hard struggle to regain a measure of independence and functionality within the limits of her physical disability.

Last Wednesday I went to clinic where they decided to order my second corset, a strong belt from the brace shop (for standing purposes, a posture panel and a crutch pocket for my [wheel]chair; feeder equipment (which means ball bearing equipment under each arm to replace lost shoulder and arm motion). I get a flying saucer under the left arm and a ball bearing feeder trough under the right. A flying saucer is a little round padded elbow support attached to a ball bearing-swivel arm, and assists one in reaching. A feeder trough is a metal cradle affair in which you rest your forearm when you are minus a biceps to bend the elbow. It is very delicately balanced and you can learn to use the helpless arm with this assistance. These are attached to the arms of the wheelchair. Also, I get double springs for my arm slings and my high lapboard needed adjusting, (which brought about the idea for the next Wheelchair Review cartoon — and to continue me on a full functional program. They commended my loss of weight (now 139) and admonished me to continue doing so.

Although I would never have thought it possible, twice last week I managed to find my balance on braces and crutches and STOOD ALONE — once for almost 10 minutes. However, I am still highly unreliable at this

113

activity — and please don't become over exuberant as this does NOT mean I will be walking. I still do not have enough power in the right side to permit movement. The purpose of the crutch balancing is to enable one to find his balance standing, thus facilitating moving him [the patient] without involving too much lifting. But each new accomplishment is a step forward! Friday with the aid of my trusty aluminum cane, I was able to pull myself over on the left side for the first time, going about it in my usual backward fashion and PUSHing with my left biceps rather than PULLing, thus dumb- founding all the P.T's.

On February 14—Valentine's Day—John and Rainie treated themselves to a phone call, apparently only the first or second since she had arrived at Warm Springs, and the first opportunity the children had had to hear their mother's voice or speak to her in months. In a letter two days later, Rainie apologized for talking so long and said she felt "very guilty for the size of the phone bill," another sign of just how tight the Clarkes' finances were. Nonetheless, Rainie continued her exhausting rehabilitation and hectic social schedule:

(February 16, 1955) I've been kept so busy this week that I haven't had time to catch my breath! I start with a wheelchair function treatment at 9:30; pool at 10 and 10:30; crutch balancing at 11:30; then lunch at Georgia Hall at 12:00. Mat at 2:30; crutch balancing at 4:00 and feeder class at 4:30 — and you can imagine what a rat race it is when you figure all the changes of clothing that accompany this routine. As soon as I have my bath in the morn I put on my bathing suit and then my corset and clothing as there isn't time before the pool to come back and change. Talk about quick change artist! All I lack is a pair of breakaway suspenders and a fright wig. And my hair is rapidly beginning to look like a fright wig as it is. Today I had to stay over in Roosevelt Hall from 2:30 until after 5 as I had to be in the brace shop from 3 to 4 while Frank Jones, one of the brace men, worked on my equipment. Then I had to rush back to the room after supper to help one of the student PTs put on a make-up for a skit

114

her class was doing at a party they are giving for the medical staff tonite. By that time, I simply gave up the ghost and went to bed. They are trying to talk me into singing a couple of blues numbers for the Fellowship meeting, this Sunday night, but I have refused.

(February 21, 1955) They pulled a dirty trick on me last nite in the theatre at Roosevelt Hall. The student PTs put on the skit I mentioned before so the patients could see it. Then afterwards Dr. Gosling played for a community sing — his last public performance as he goes back to Walter Reed Friday. After the first few numbers Viv Erickson (the blonde PT, who asked us if we knew some of her friends in Ridgewood — and who seems to MC most of the affairs hereabouts) announced to the audience that there was someone In the audience who could sing blues and wouldn't they like to hear her - whereupon I was forcibly dragged up on the stage and therewith rendered, "A Good Man Is Hard To Find", "St. Louis Blues" and "Frivolous Sal", with the spotlights et al. The best I can say is that I created considerable noise for a respirator case — although I have had several favorable comments. Over the week-end I wrote a special material number which Dr. Gosling has promised to help me set the [to?] music to tonite.[6] (I'm requiring my pound of flesh for that double dealing last nite).

In fact, in addition to the many other social activities Rainie was engaged in, she found time to send each of the three children an on-going series of illustrated children's stories, each tailored to one of the children. Toby's was the story of "Miss Flutterby," a butterfly. Chris received stories about "Beauregard Beatle," so named undoubtedly because he had "been" Beauregard, Elsie the Borden cow's son. And little Timmy, only now going on four years old, received the tales of "Anthony Ant." Unfortunately, all but one of these beautifully written and illustrated stories have been lost, but they reflected Rainie's skills as an artist as well as her effort to reach out and "touch" her children while so far away.

[6.] The "special material number" was called "The Dowager's Lament." See text box, next page.

The Dowager's Lament
(or "The Season's Not the Season Any More")
By
Rainie Clarke

When I lift my lorgnette
at the opening of the Met,
and I spy a lady's feet upon the table not the floor;
When I take my Pekingese
for a stroll to catch the breeze
and she stops to sniff that perfect little mongrel from next door;
When I take my friends to tea
at the dear Old Colony
and I find it's full of chorus girls galore,
Well, it's very clear to me
things aren't what they used to be
and the season's not "The Season" anymore.

When I go to Epsom Downs
and they're wearing short-length gowns
and they've asked a gay divorcee if she wouldn't like to pour;
When I winter at Palm Beach,
I am quite bereft of speech
at the strangest kind of people who are cluttering up the shore;
When I'm studying *Who's Who*
and I find the blood's not blue
and it's full of peasants one should just ignore,
Well, I've certainly demonstrated
that the season's overrated
and the season's not "The Season" anymore.

When I'm visiting El Cid
or the bull ring in Madrid
and I find a lady fighting like a common matador;
When I'm riding to the hounds
and the fox gets out of bounds
and "the hunt" forgets to shout their "Yoikes" and "Tally Hos"
    before;
When *Burke's Peerage* I peruse
and I find there simply slews of people who made money from the
    War,
though I hardly dare to say so

116

you can bet your bottom *peso*
that the season's not "The Season" anymore.

When I'm basking in the sand
of the Riviera strand
and the girls' attire is just a brief suggestion aft and fore;
When I'm playing at roulette
and the one to place a bet
is an ex-Egyptian Pharaoh with his arm around a wh---- lady!;
When the Almanac de Gotha
Can't be sampled any fahther
by the princess of the five-and-ten cent store,
You can bet your bottom *lire*
that it couldn't be any clearer
that the season's not "The Season" anymore.

When I find a rusty spot
on the railing of my yacht
and the ash trays in my Rolls are overflowing on the floor;
When the income from my trust
isn't strictly "upper crust"
and the coupons that I clip
are not as gilt-edged as of yore;
When my diamond tiara
must be hocked so I can borrow
enough to pay for my Canasta score;
When a Social Pedigree
can't compare with A.K.C.
then the season's not "The Season" anymore, Dear me!
the season's not "The Season" anymore.

When I'm sporting cashmere knits
on the slopes of St. Moritz
and my guide turns out to be the one who *didn't* teach the Shah;
When I'm feeling very hearty
at the Elsa Maxwell party
and I find my dinner partner's an unmitigated bore;
When the waiter doesn't warn ya
that the wine's from California
and the caviar's the kind you just deplore;
You can bet your bottom crown
that the world is upside down
And the season's not "The Season" anymore.

117

When I decorate my belly
with a gown by Schiaparelli
and I find I should have bought my things from Christian Dior;
When the moths invade my villa
and devour my best chinchilla
and they tell me Harry Winston can't produce the Koh-I-Noor;
When I see the Claridge fade
and the lack of carriage trade
and they don't know what a marriage is made for;
You can bet your bottom pound
I have definitely found
that the season's not "The Season" anymore.

When I am no longer showered
by the wit of Mr. Coward
and the season doesn't offer anything by Mr. Shaw;
When I'm faced with the decision
to stay home with television
since there isn't any opening that can boast a Barrymore;
Shall I watch the Brooklyn Dodgers
or hear Hammerstein and Rogers
both of whom, I must admit, I just adore;
You can bet your bottom *sou*
or your tickets to "Talu"
that the season's not "The Season" anymore, more's the pity,
the Social Season's definitely through!

When I patronize the Derby
and I'm photographed by Zerbe
and the picture in *The Tattler* shows the house instead of me;
When I look just like a creation
in my shot by Cecil Beaton
and it fills my social rivals with a catty kind of glee;
When I can't get any closer
to a wife of Rubirosa
than the woman who is sitting next to me;
You can bet your bottom *franc*
that the social season stank
and it's nothing like "The Season" ought to be.

When my friends are all employed
in a bout with Mr. Freud,

and they wander in dejected like the Dane of Elsinore;
When the Knickerbocker's "Cholly"
snubs the Duke and Dahling Wally,
and Monaco's just a country on the North African shore,
When I can't catch barracuda
off the coast of dear Bermuda
and the Stork is just a bird that knows the score;
Then I'll definitely know
that it's really, truly so
and the season's not "The Season" anymore. Oh, well!
The Social Season's finally shot to Hell!

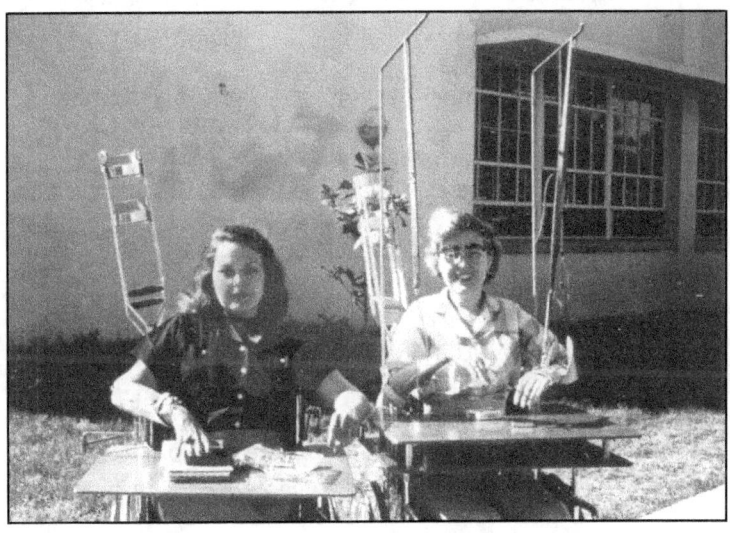

Rainie and another patient at the Georgia Warm Springs
Foundation, Spring 1955.

Meanwhile...back at the ranch

While Rainie was working hard and enjoying the camaraderie of the Warm Springs "family," her family back home was having a difficult time. John obviously hesitated to share his troubles with Rainie, but it is clear from his letters to her that the constant worry, especially the financial pressure, and the necessity of taking care of three small children while trying to find enough work to make ends meet, were taking a toll on him — both physically and emotionally. In a February 23 letter to Rainie, the dam finally broke:

> Never have I been so ashamed of myself — and I have no good reason or excuse to offer — I JUST HAVEN'T WRITTEN for so long that I feel terribly about it. Everyday I think, well, I'll get to it today — and then I don't. I'm afraid I've been pretty ambitionless and downright lazy in addition to not feeling quite up to snuff...
>
> Last week I wracked my brain and imagination trying to raise $150 so we could leave last Friday and visit you for a few days. Even MY imagination wouldn't stretch THAT far. I guess I told you that the youngsters had this week as MID [winter] vacation and I thought it was the ideal time to DO SOMETHING. I even thought that when we could afford to come down there we might try to go to [his half-sister] Wanna, since it was so much closer and there'd be no living expenses. JUST ANYTHING TO BREAK THIS DAMNED MONOTONY. Then the more I thought about it the more I decided it would be pretty silly. If they were really interested in us Wanna would have come here long ago (if only for a day or two) and it was kinda silly for me to go running to her — SO we've done NOTHING. It has been the most depressing weather this past week that anyone could even dream of. Rain, fog, smirk [sic.] or dark damp drizzling depressing days since the middle of last week. [After taking the children to another couple's house for dinner], I had another MISERABLE stomach ache so we stopped at a drug store in Hohokus for a bottle of bisodol.

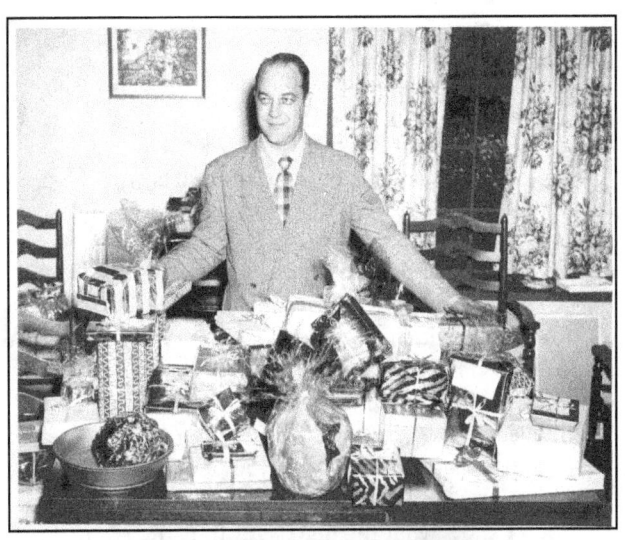

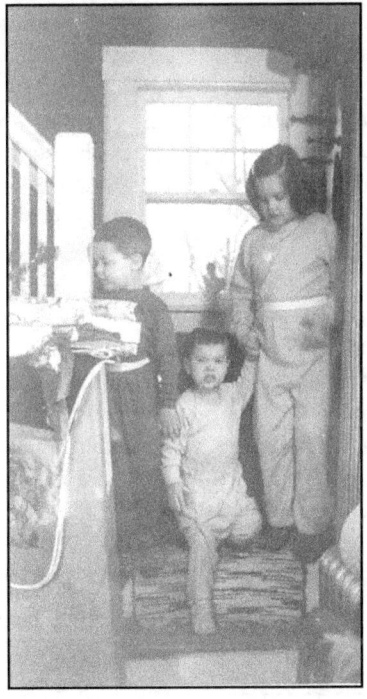

Christmas 1953 (top) and 1954 (bottom) when Rainie was in the hospital. Notice how fatigued John looks in the top picture. The bountiful Christmases were mostly the result of the benevolence of friends and the community.

With the hot water bottle I finally got to sleep a little after 2 and slept fitfully till 6.[7]

Again a week or so later, John showed how much the strain was affecting him:

(March 1, 1955) Sweetheart, Girl:

Are you ever going to forgive me? Do you realize it has been, OVER two weeks since I wrote you? In fact, our phone conversation on Valentines Day was our last communication ... except for the niteletter [telegram] last Saturday night, which I hope you understood.

I don't know what the hell has gotten into me unless it is as I said "a full-of-the-moon-spell". I don't seem to be able to think, get started, do, plan — or even just sit still. Guess I NEED YOU! — always have said I wasn't worth a damn without you to tell we what to do and when to do it and how to do it. Could you possibly send me one of your HOW-TO-DO-IT kits? — or DO-IT-YOURSELF instruction sheetz? Truth of the matter I think I'm in my MENOPAUSE — and more pause than man.

There I go, doing exactly what I would have done if is why I didn't write because of!!! [sic.] Truthfully it is pretty hard to settle down (I really mean get STARTED into) a letter in that frame of mind. You wonder what the hell you can say, spend a long time trying to think of SOMETHING and wind up with NOTHING and still not fooling ANYONE — so everyday "tomorrow I gotta" and then don't. You know, seriously, very little happens when you just sit on your big fat dairyair, to write about. Except for dinner on G. Wash Bday [George Washington's birthday] and two trips into town I haven't been out of the house in over a month

---

[7.] It is unclear whether this was more than merely a stomach ache exacerbated by worry. John a few years later would have an emergency gall bladder surgery and within a few more years, a heart attack. These pains may have been the early warning signs of either problem.

except to dash to Grand Union, [the grocery store] around
the corner and back - so what's to write about? ME?
(horsestuff) — the YOUNGSTERS? (the little basquets) —
or a damned dirty, EMPTY house?

When he could, and when the mental funk lifted a little,
John often sought refuge in hard work outside:

Friday turned out to be a fairly decent day, pretty warm
and beautifully sunshiny all day — so I got AMBITIOUS —
you know me, there's nothing like getting my hands in
dirt. I had allowed the youngsters to play ON THE PATHS,
down in the back, to the bridge. I saw them TRYING to
straddle limbs of that big old tree that lays just beyond the
gate, pretending [to ride] horses. I went down to try to
better that situation. Consequently I spent all day Friday,
Saturday and yesterday working my fanny off down in the
back. All I've been able to think of since is "wish Mommy
was here so she could see this".

Except for back up in the hole where the stumps and crap
is I have that whole area, from the path to the bottom
of the right-of-way and from the gate to the small creek all
clear and burned off. I left the berry bushes to the left of
the path so that we might have a few berries if you get
home in time this summer. On the other side I cleaned
out all the briars, weeds, trash and stuff. In doing so I
found about three nice young trees which I cleaned up
and left — the willow and a couple of others. I trimmed
off the big old fallen tree and made three different limbs
on it as horses for our three cowBOYS (trimmed some of
the bark for saddles etc) and they've had the time of their
sweet young lives down there since.

Sunday was a nasty day and we didn't get out at all but I
worked down there all day again yesterday and have it all
finished down to the little creek. In many instances I was
able to pull the roots of the berry bushes so they won't be
springing right back up again. I have worked like a dog.
BUT it has helped clear my mind a little and get me back to
some "right thinking" which I needed damned badly.

123

Yesterday morning I took time off from outdoors to get a million little things done that have been bothering me. Fixing one of the hinges on the top bunk bed which "just got splitted", a knob and hinge on the change chest, which "just fell off", a rip in the nursery linoleum, which "a ghost did", a couple of hooks in Toby's room and the same in our closet, a coat of paint on a couple of picture frames, one of those small framed mirrors securely screwed to the back of the bathroom door for the boys to "see IF their faces are clean" and so on and so on.

Times were not always so grim at the Clarkes', however. While writing Rainie a letter, apparently in March, John closed as follows:

Good Gawd, the boys just got up and you have never heard such whoopin' and hollerin' and carryin' on in your life. They're both in good mood but full of ── and vinegar — both hanging over my shoulders yelling "TELL MOMMY WE LOOOOVE HER" — "GIVE MOMMY OUR KISSES" — "MAKE A WHOLE BUNCH OF KISSES ON THERE" — then running around chasing each other in circles here in the kitchen.

Just gotta stop and DO something with them — whoops, there went a dog right on top of the typewriter. They CAN be a lot of fun when they wake up like this and are extra nice.

Remember we all love you to pieces and miss you the same way. We ALL send bushels of kisses and acres of hugs.

Returning home

By February, John and Rainie were beginning to think about and plan for her eventual return. It was uncertain at that point whether she would be able to return directly home or would have to stay in a local rehabilitation facility for some time. They were exploring both options. John talked with local officials about the

124

possibility of assistance from the New Jersey State Rehabilitation Center after Rainie returned from Warm Springs, but apparently nothing came of it.

For her part, Rainie was thinking big. In late February, she shared some of her potential plans—or, at least, hopes—with John:

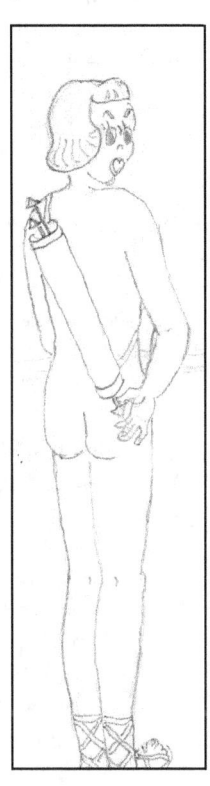

At lunch today I was talking to a girl at my table who had been an art student and we happened to mention that Famous Artist Course that I was interested in last summer. She said that Mrs. Freyman, the psychologist, had told her that quite often the State Rehabilitation Committee would finance courses like that — also last nite Ruth Nimey and I were fooling around the piano in Georgia Hall (when no one was around) and I feel that with a suspension sling on my right arm I could manage to play again — at least enough to accompany myself. So, if the opportunity presents itself I shall investigate the possibility of State Rehabilitation subsidizing either an art course or a music course. Just think I might be a flaming success yet!!

Just think of the emotional impact of rolling into an agent's office in full regalia and equipment and asking point blank for a job!! How could they refuse you?? Of course you realize the extent of my facetiousness - but I can DREAM, can't I?

Sketch of a female Cupid by Rainie done at Warm Springs, 1954-55.

In mid-March, Rainie described the advanced occupational therapy program she was attending, a program that deeply appealed to her artistic side.

I went to clinic last Monday - didn't learn anything new —
just keep up with the same program but add OT, occupational therapy, which I started this week. Have already
discovered that I can operate a sewing machine
successfully — and am in the midst of making an oven
mitt. I told my OT (Occupational Therapist) that I want to
learn ceramics and jewelry making (metal), both of which I
feel I could operate successfully at home in a limited
amount of space (particularly jewelry) and I think there
would be a commercial outlet for both in Ridgewood and
environs. You can see I'm considering all the creative
money-making schemes possible — I am determined to be
a contributing force one way or another.

She was also thinking hard about how the house could be
rearranged so she could play a full role as mother, wife, and housekeeper:

We really should start thinking about necessary changes
to be made in the house — I find each day, more and
more things I will be able to do provided the appliances
are accessible — and the house, what they refer to as
"functional". Of course many of their ideas are
theoretically fine but financially impossible — however I
wish I could convince you of my still firm conviction that
remodeling the basement is the most practical answer to
our problems. And of course, the ideal time to make
changes would be while I'm still hospitalized — but
obviously that's financially out of the question right now.

I see people going home every week and judging by their
various conditions and abilities, I don't think it will be too
many more months before I shall be ready to come home.
Right now I'm putting my powers of concentration to work
on the acquisition of a Ted Hoyer hoist — a gadget
designed to lift a patient to and from various places,
including car and bathtub — thereby saving your back. I
am continuing to lose weight — now 133 — but that's still
quite a chunk to lift in and out of a tub. The hoist sells for
$265.00, with bathtub attachment, which is why I'm

concentrating! I also have several ideas of my own, which I am sure you will be able to enlarge upon and perfect — including a work table on casters with drop leaf arms and on which I would be able to use the sewing machine, the ironer, typewriter etc... I think by attaching a long lever to the ironer control, I will be able to operate the ironer — also with a pair of "reachers" with rubber tips, I believe I can operate the washer. I've already surprised myself with how well I can get into the refrigerator, including the freezer compartment — unless ours proves to be much higher than this one. I can also manage some things at the stove provided they aren't too heavy — my limitations are still in the matter of lifting and reaching — but my endurance continues to improve.

Rainie was not, of course, the only seriously affected polio patient at Warm Springs, nor the only one with big ideas. In April. she described one of her companions and a would-be co-author:

Yvonne Hudson, a very sweet gal from Winnipeg and I have collaborated on several good ideas for mystery novels — the first of which is a golfing mystery entitled "Hole in One". The only trouble is that just about half the foundation has heard about it — and every time we get together to TRY to do a little serious work — at least five or six other people roll into Yvonne's room where we usually work, to hear the thing progress, and it winds up a free-for-all with very little getting accomplished. They all seem to feel it's a new kind of game.

We have to work fast as Yvonne is leaving in a couple of weeks — so we're hoping to have the plot outline, sequence of events, character and motivation finished by the time she leaves — then I will work on manuscript and mail it to her for revisions. If the experiment proves successful we hope eventually to invest in a tape recorder and electric typewriter for Yvonne. You see, Yvonne's arms and hands are completely involved — she uses feeder equipment with T-bars and feeds herself, puts on her lipstick — with the aid of a mouth stick she turns

127

pages In her books — and even managed to write a letter with it one day.

She's quite a remarkable gal, and incidentally, quite beautiful. She feels that she could type on an electric typewriter with a mouth stick — and we could communicate our ideas by tape recorder since our ideas seem to germinate thru talking them out.

Finally, in May, the time had come. John packed the children into the car and drove from New Jersey to Georgia, a wonderful adventure for the children, but no doubt a trying time for John. Staying in a local boarding house, the children explored the unfamiliar surroundings[8] while John attended numerous briefings and familiarization sessions with the PTs, OTs, and nurses, learning how Rainie's equipment worked, what her capabilities and limitations were, and how best to approach such tasks as getting her into and out of bed, wheelchair, car, and bathtub, how to attend to her intimate needs, and how to move her around in bed to change linens, etc. After a few short days, the family headed back up the road to await Rainie's arrival by airplane.

[8.] Among other things, Chris and Tim enjoyed exploring the crawl space under the raised house, a filthy area where the host family's cats liked to escape the Georgia heat—and probably a sometime lair of snakes and other dangerous creatures. Chris, then about six, also remembers learning to whistle during his stay at the boarding house, a discovery that no doubt drove everyone else crazy as he persistently practiced a tuneless imitation of a real whistle.

Following pages: Photos of Warm Springs Foundation,
early 1950s from official postcards.

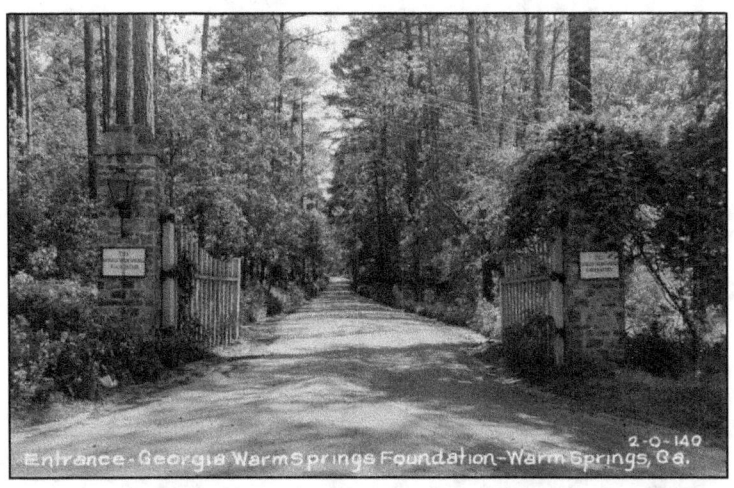

Entrance - Georgia Warm Springs Foundation - Warm Springs, Ga.   2-0-140

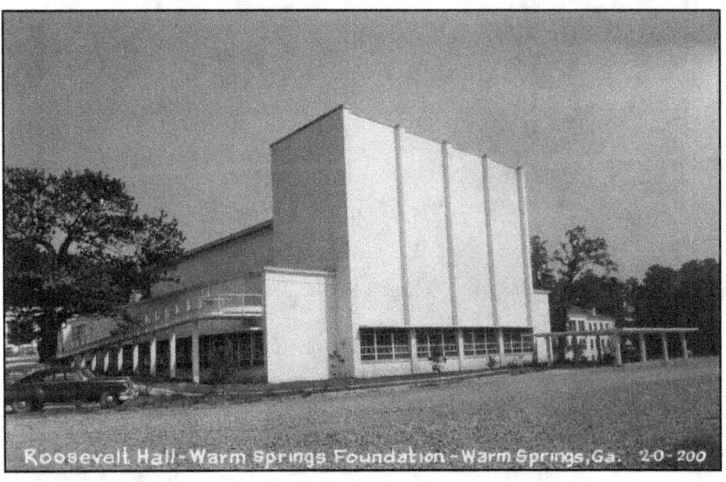

Roosevelt Hall - Warm Springs Foundation - Warm Springs, Ga.   2-0-200

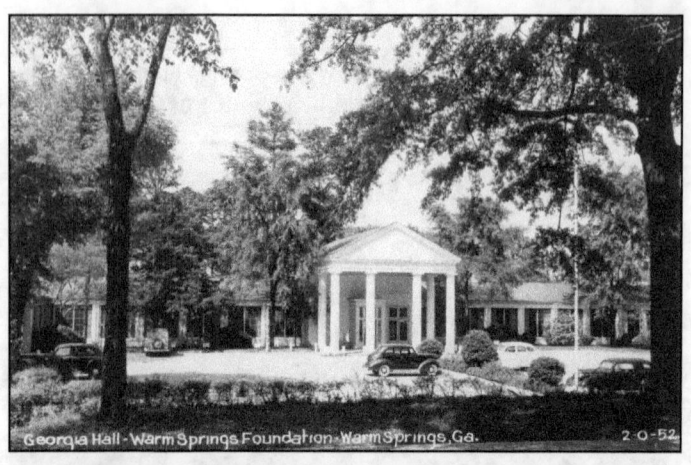

Georgia Hall - Warm Springs Foundation - Warm Springs, Ga.   2-0-52

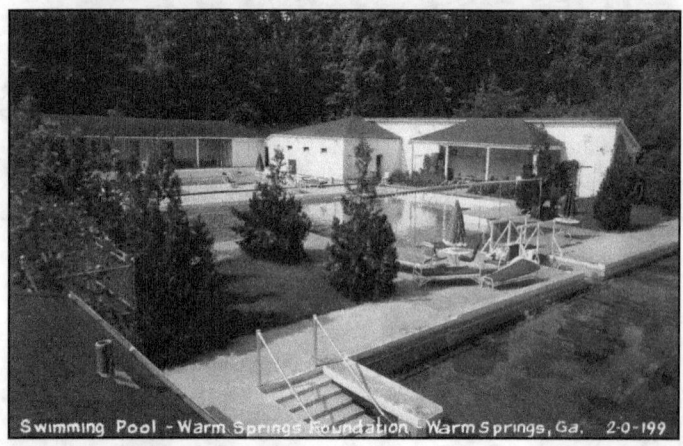

Swimming Pool - Warm Springs Foundation - Warm Springs, Ga.   2-0-199

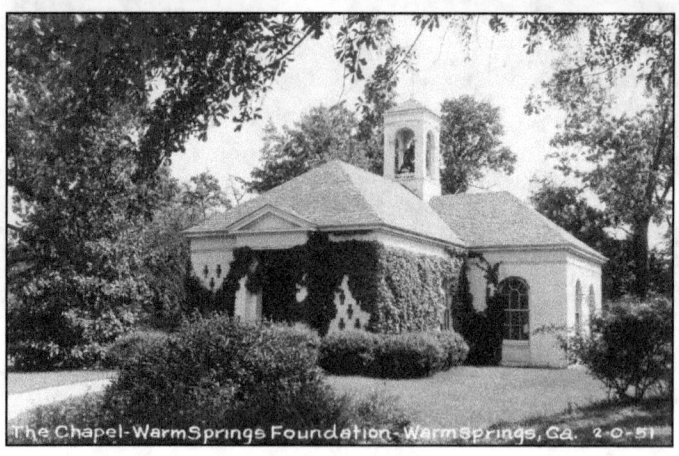

The Chapel - Warm Springs Foundation - Warm Springs, Ga.   2-0-51

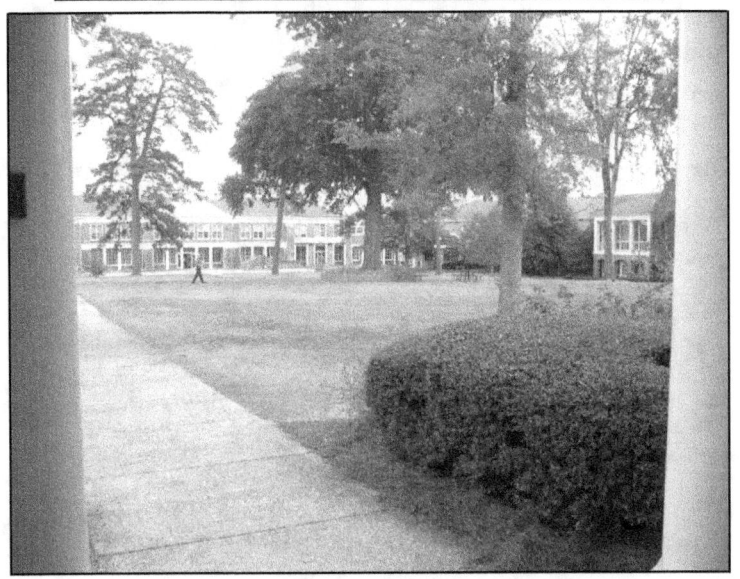

Central Quadrangle.

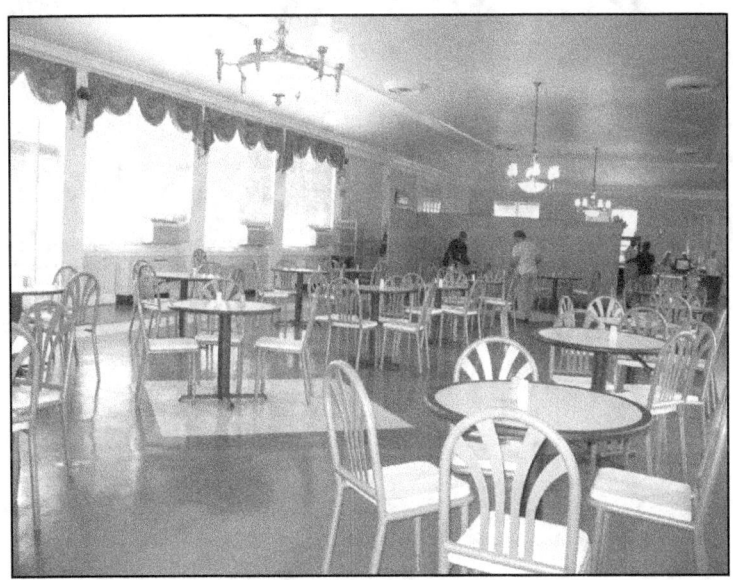

Old Dining Room.

131

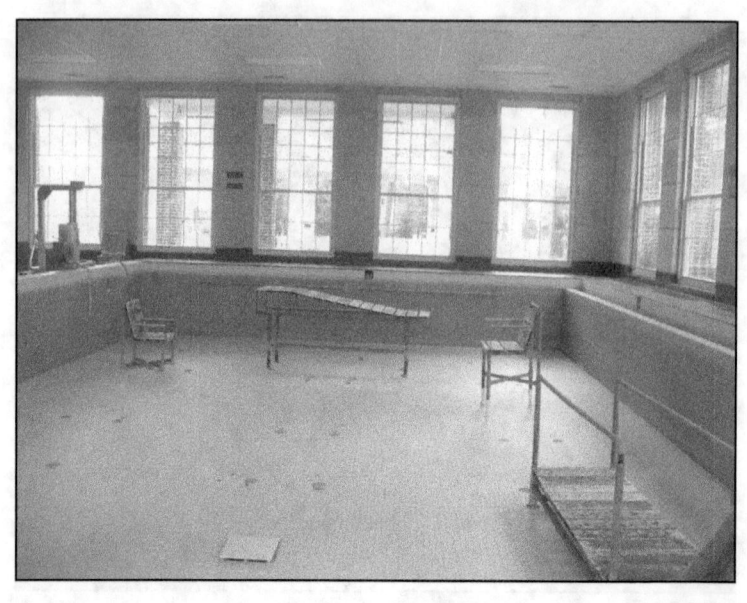

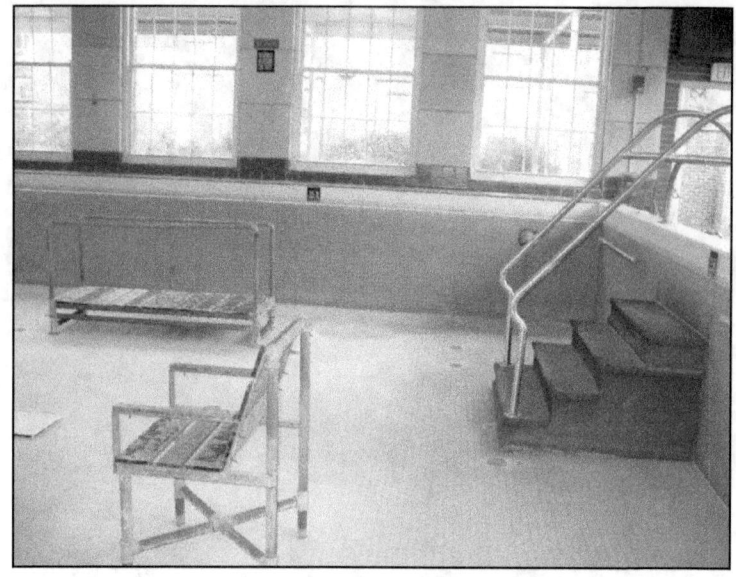

Old therapy pool, no longer used.

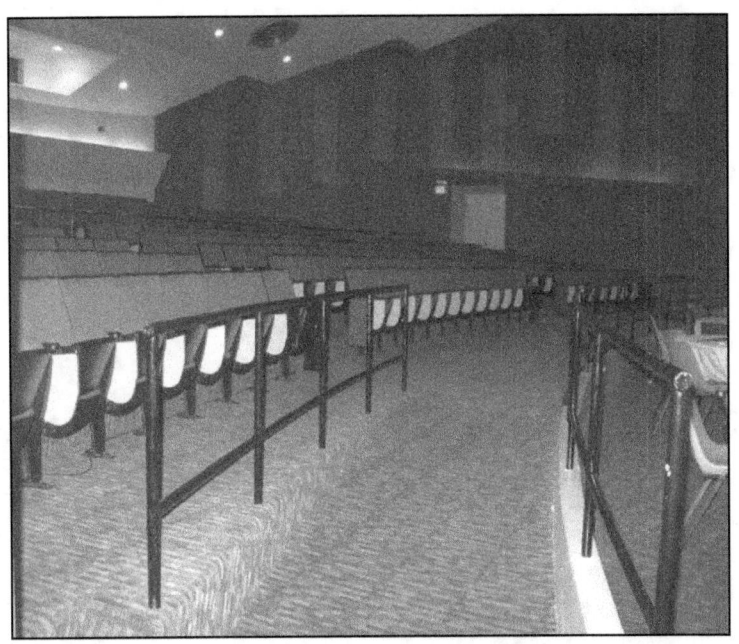

Theater.

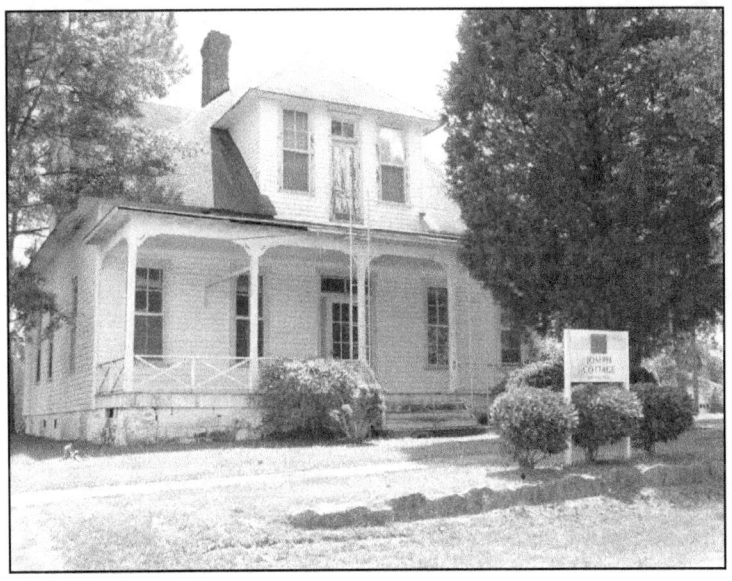

One of the old staff cottages, now being restored.

Split-level Schizophrenia— Life Returns to "Normal"

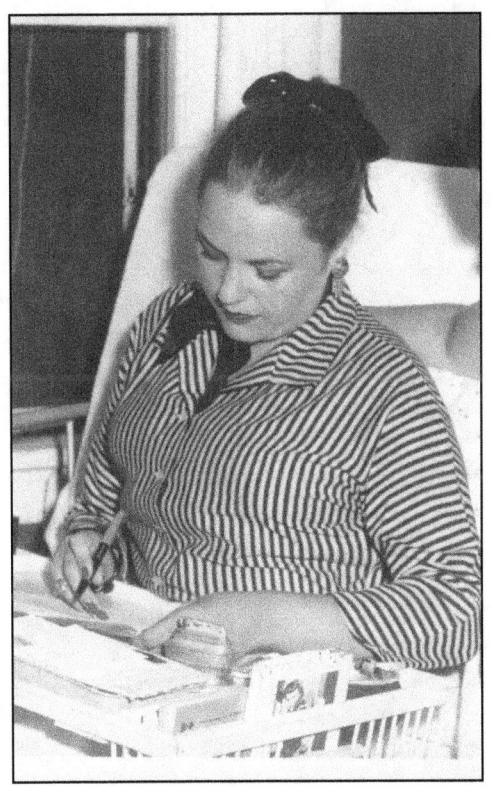

Previous page: Photo of Rainie Clarke signing a voter's registration card in 1956 or 1957. She was permitted to sign the card at home.

Happy Landings
By
Rainie Clarke

The lap of God is covered with a patchwork quilt. I leaned my head against the window of the plane and looked down at the countryside spread out below me; squares of brown and rust, green and black, oblongs, rectangles, semi-circles, laced with winding ribbons of blue and amber. Viewed from the right perspective, the lap of God becomes the lap of luxury. I squeezed my thoughts back to that present moment. I had left Warm Springs, Georgia far behind me and I was going home.

The stewardess brought my lunch. She smiled. "How are you traveling, Mrs. Clarke ?"

"Oh, fine. Wonderfully!"

"Would you like for me to cut your meat?"

"If you please. I'm at a disadvantage without my chair."

"Is there anything else I can do?" she asked.

"If you'll kindly place the coffee on my left? I've become a southpaw."

I surveyed the meal. It looked delightful, but at that moment I think bread and water would have looked like sumptuous fare to me.

In a surprisingly short time the stewardess was announcing, "We are flying over Philadelphia. We will land at Newark airport in sixteen minutes."

Excitement bubbled up inside me like ginger ale. My family had spent a full week with me just seven days before in what might be considered my graduation exercises from the Georgia Warm Springs Foundation. That was the first time I had seen them in six months. It combined a period of family counseling and gay holiday in the rarified atmosphere of rehabilitation hospital and winter resort that distinguishes the fabulous Foundation from any other place on earth.

But this was different. This was coming home! I faced the immediate present with joy and a certain amount of stage fright. My doubts about the future I parked behind my chewing gum and glanced at the blinking sign ahead of me.

"Fasten your seat belts." I smiled to myself. "That won't be necessary. Mine's been fastened since we took off from Atlanta." The other passengers began to stir in the anticipation of landing. Suddenly the plane gave a gentle bounce, the wheels kissed the runway and we taxied to the smooth finale of what had been an incredibly short trip.

Passengers studded the aisle like mushrooms; then roved slowly forward to disembark through the hatch which was directly opposite my seat. I intercepted several glances which said, very obviously, "What the devil is she sitting there for? Doesn't she know this is the end of the line?" And two or three sets of feminine eyes registered dismay or outright horror as they took in my red denim pedal pushers.

I was not affected. I felt wonderful. I knew I looked better than I had in years. I had shed some seventy pounds in the last eighteen months. I might not be very functional, but I had one arm, two hands, I could breathe, my mascara was on straight, and I was GOING HOME!

As the flight steward picked me up, my mind flashed back six months to my exit from the plane in Atlanta on my way to Warm Springs. I had been carried out on a draw sheet by four men, two of the airline's personnel and two ambulance attendants. The stewardess brought up the rear. Well, not exactly. She brought up the feet. The rear played a merry little tune of accompaniment as it bumped every step on the way down by itself. I decided that if my rebirth into the world of normalcy had to be in the breech position, at least I was lucky that I wasn't dragging my keel.

John stood at the foot of the steps taking snap shots of the whole performance. Later, after they were developed, he gazed at the pictures with a look of tragic disappointment and remarked that it was really too bad he hadn't brought along a bottle of champagne for the occasion. I could see what he meant. The flight steward looked wonderful, but my posterior, being the nearest thing to the camera, had assumed abnormally wide proportions. Just the same, I resolved to learn to spit as my only adequate means of defense against his bright remarks.

And so, Rainie returned to the home she had only lived in for two months. John had made a number of changes to accommodate Rainie's return and her needs. There was no question of her returning to her second floor bedroom; tending to her would have been more difficult and she would have been isolated, with the kitchen, family room, and dining room on the first floor. So John had turned the sun porch into a bedroom for Rainie.

The sun porch was small, about eight-by-ten feet, with three sides entirely occupied by windows. There was no door, only a large vaulted entryway. While this facilitated moving equipment in and out of the room, it meant there was no built-in privacy. John had heavy curtains hung across the three sides of the room and the entryway, all on sliding rails, so during the day Rainie could look out into the front yard and see the woods (the third side was behind the head of her bed), while at night, the curtains could be drawn across the windows and entrance. When attending to her private needs, the curtains could also be drawn, rendering her room a nice, private "nest."

For the first year or so after her return, John would sometimes get Rainie up, either using the Hoyer hoist or simply lifting her from bed to wheelchair. He had installed a ramp from the front door, so she could go outside in nice weather, and even take rides in the car. In fact, the very night she arrived home, they went to a party so Rainie could meet some of the town folk and, hopefully, resume the active social life she had always enjoyed. As with so many aspects of life, however, attending this party became a story, part comedy, part farce, with a tinge of tragedy and pathos mixed in:

The Party
By
Rainie Clarke

[On the way home from the airport], John reached over and patted my hand. "It's good to have you home, honey!" he said. "By the way, do you feel like going to a party tonight ? We have an invitation." "Of course I do. Where ?" "The Marble Hill Civic Theater group is having an after-theater party.[1] I thought it would be a good way for you to meet some people in town. You know hardly anybody. Do you think you'll feel up to it ?"

"Certainly she will," interposed Meadows.[2] ""We'll put her to bed when we get home. She can rest until time to dress for the party."

"What time is the party?" I asked, not sure that John and Meadows realized how much time the dressing process required.

"Eleven-thirty. It's at the Algonquin Inn." Pappy replied.

I began to anticipate the obstacles. "How do we get in ?" I inquired. "It's perfectly simple," said Pappy, "There are only about four steps. I'll take the chair up first. Then I'll carry you in and put you in it."

The practical problems having been settled, I began to feel like Cinderella after the fairy-godmother said she could go to the ball.

The Cinderella bit was not too far-fetched. Godmother Meadows and I decided on a dress I had bought two years before but had never worn. It was a cocktail length pure silk organdy,

---

[1] This story was part of an autobiography in which Rainie had changed the name of the town, locations, and people. I have left it as she wrote it, not attempting to reconstruct the actual names or locations. "Marble Hill," however, was the code-name for Ridgewood.

[2] "Meadows" was a live-in aide for Rainie whose employment had been arranged by the National Foundation for Infantile Paralysis. See pages 159-161.

changing, according to lights, from green to purple. I was adamant about not wearing my little red ground grippers.

"What am I going to do for shoes?" I wailed. "I can't wear high heels. They make my ankles wobble. I can't go barefooted, and I *won't* wear those red oxfords with that dress!" John, who is equal to almost any problem, bounded up the stairs, returning in a few minutes with a pair of black velvet and silver kid mules.

"How about these?" he smiled. "Just the thing," said Meadows. "There's only a strap across the instep. They'll be easy to get on and off and the heels aren't too high." It's so comforting to have a husband of superior intelligence. Cinderella Clarke was ready to step out.

For a man in show business, John is abnormally reticent about "making entrances". He likes to enter and leave places as unobtrusively as possible. Unfortunately it is not possible to unload and assemble sixty-eight pounds of equipment and one hundred thirty pounds of wife unobtrusively. In the first place, little groups of people begin to gather like flies around a kitchen door, anxious to help. Various individuals start grabbing the smaller items such as posture panel, seat cushion, feeder arms, lap board, ash tray and my pocket-book and begin trailing in and out of wherever we happen to be going like safari ants. (It is an interesting phenomenon that John is always left to wrestle the sixty-four pound chair and the one hundred thirty pound wife by himself.)

In the second place, it seems to hold all the fascination of unloading the circus, attracting a considerable crowd of slack-jawed, open-mouthed sidewalk superintendents. Unless we develop Commando tactics of arriving only after midnight on moonless nights, I assume that our arrivals and departures will continue to be attended by all the curiosity seekers within a ten mile radius. Pappy has finally accepted the fact that wherever we go from now on, we shall arrive and depart about as unobtrusively as the *Queen Elizabeth*.

The Algonquin Inn is a pre-Revolutionary War structure, remodeled into a charming restaurant and cocktail lounge. It has a long and interesting history and, like so many places in Northern New Jersey, is, I presume, one of the sites where George Washington slept, ate, or rinsed out his undies. (Some people we knew many years ago bought a very old farm house near Tenafly. They claimed a singular distinction for their home. They stated that it was the only house in Bergen county over a hundred years old where George Washington had *never* slept. Judging by the wonderful parties they threw, I do not believe anybody ever slept there.)

Be that as it may, the Algonquin Inn was displaying a rugged constitution and no symptoms of advanced senility, when, at nearly midnight, we swept up the circular driveway and parked at the front door.

Pappy had underestimated the steps. Six stone steps led up to the door, with two more inside leading to the foyer. As John made the frequent trips into the building to arrange and assemble my chair, I thought of the childhood story—"and another little ant took another grain of wheat and put it in the pile, and another little ant.."

John returned to carry me in, while the doorman stood by, twittering in helpless anxiety. We started up the stairs and my right slipper fell off. I whispered, "I thought the part called for losing a slipper on the way out."

John set me down in the chair, retrieving the slipper from the doorman who was obviously delighted to be of some service. John put the slipper back on my foot, adjusted the arm supports and lap board and looked in the bar for a familiar face.

Just then an ethereal blonde floated down the narrow, thickly carpeted staircase. She saw John and greeted him in traditional civic theater language. "Dahling!" John turned to me and said, "Honey, I want you to meet Gwendolyn Cloverdale." We gave each other a quick feminine appraisal as Pappy said, "Where's the crowd ?"

Gwendolyn looked distressed. "Dahling, I'm so sorry," she said. "The plans were changed at the last minute. The party's upstairs in the private dining room." Pappy heaved a sigh, grabbed a straight chair and transferred me to it. By then I was beginning to feel less and less like Cinderella and more and more like a French bed doll, with arms and legs flopping in all directions.

Pappy carried up the chair and most of the other equipment (which sounds pretty simple; however each move requires dismantling and folding the chair, then unfolding and reassembling it at the point of destination). He came back down lighting a cigarette, pulled up a chair and sat down to rest for a minute.

"Get ready for a long haul," he said. "There are ten steps to the landing, ten more steps to the second floor, then two steps up to the dining room—all steep."

"Wouldn't it be simpler to carry me up over your shoulder in a kind of fireman's rescue hold?" I asked. John said, "Not the way my stomach's hurting. My gall bladder's kicking up again."

I looked at him. He had turned a saffron yellow.

"Oh, honey, let's just send up our regrets and go home." I said.

"Absolutely not," John answered. "We said we were going and we are. We're going to have a good time if it kills me." John is nothing if not determined.

He asked Gwendolyn to follow us, picked me up and started up the stairs. Half way up the first flight, my right slipper fell off. Gwendolyn caught it. Half way up the second flight, my left slipper fell off. Gwendolyn caught it. We finally made the second floor, where he set me down in the chair. As he leaned over to replace the slippers, he muttered, "The next time you wear shoes like these, I'm going to pin them to your garter belt."

"As parties go this one was not spectacular. The room was too small to accommodate the horseshoe table. A sit-down affair such as this one turned out to be limits your contact to your immediate neighbors, unless you go in for hog-calling. My immediate neighbors happened to be people I had already met. I was, of course, delighted to see them again, but I did not have an opportunity to meet any of the fifty or sixty people whom I did not know.

Before we left home, John had warned me that our finances were in their usual state of jeopardy and suggested that I go light on ordering. I settled for glass of sherry which is my favorite social beverage anyway. We did meet, briefly a couple who were later to mean a great deal to us, Doctor Kenneth Byington and his wife, Barbara.[3]

We discovered another obstacle to party-going which we had not anticipated. Should we leave first, thereby causing a chaotic jumble of unsolicited assistance, or, at the risk of good party etiquette, wait till the bitter end to avoid the circus-striking production? We waited till the party broke up. On the way downstairs, both slippers fell off. Giddy with fatigue, I giggled, "Never mind, honey, if you wait till the clock strikes three, I'll turn into a pumpkin and roll home."

---

[3] "Dr. and Mrs. Byington" were actually Dr. Irving Selikoff and his wife, Celia. Dr. Selikoff was on his way to becoming director of the Mount Sinai school of medicine and was a pioneer in the study of the effects of asbestos on human lung tissue. His research linked the mineral to an alarmingly high risk of serious lung damage (known as asbestosis), as well as lung cancer, mesothelioma, and other cancers. As the data mounted, Dr. Selikoff became known as one of the most prominent and outspoken researchers on asbestos-related health disorders. When Dr. Selikoff took on the asbestos industry and brought to light the health crises faced by its workers, he faced intense opposition not only from the industry itself, but also from the media. He was attacked for making exaggerated claims against asbestos. Rumors even began to circulate that he had faked his medical degree.

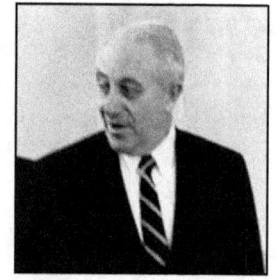

By the 1980s, however, Dr. Selikoff appeared vindicated as the tide of public opinion shifted against asbestos. Tens of thousands of sick (cont.)

Rainie's limited outings could prove both difficult and sometimes embarrassing. Having returned home in May, by July 4, she was anxious to go out and see the local fireworks display. Dutifully, John packed her in the car, along with the three youngsters who were allowed to stay up for the rare treat. In an act of thoughtlessness that was never forgotten by her young children, however, the outing was to be nearly ruined by a volunteer directing traffic at the site of the gala:

> We pulled alongside the man who was directing traffic. John leaned across me to ask him where we should park. "Officer Schultz said we should tell you we had a reservation." The man adjusted his legion cap and reckoned my wheel-chair in the "back-back" [of the station wagon]. He hocked and spat through a space in his teeth. "Pull up in the front row." He gestured ahead of us. "He raised his megaphone and shouted, "One cripple coming up!"

> Strained silence flooded the car. The kind of silence which is louder than noise. The silence where people are trying to pretend they have not heard what, obviously, they have all heard only too well.

(cont.) asbestos workers brought claims against the industry, and many won. In the 1980s, a government-mandated clean-up program in the U.S. led to massive asbestos removal projects in schools and office buildings. Even in 1955, before this party, Dr. Selikoff had been one of eight doctors jointly awarded the prestigious Albert Lasker Clinical Medical Research Award for establishing the great efficacy of isoniazid drugs in the treatment of tuberculous meningitis and generalized miliary tuberculosis. He also received awards from the American Public Health Association, the New York Academy of Sciences, and the American Cancer Society. Even at the age of 75, he continued to research the effects of asbestos. He died on May 20, 1992. Dr. Selikoff, a friend of polio pioneer Jonas Salk, in addition to being a good friend of the family, was instrumental in assuring that Rainie was put in touch with the best specialists on polio and post-polio rehabilitation. The Clarke children used to love having Celia visit because her hair—almost always worn in a bun—was long enough to reach well below her belt when unwound. Naturally, we always tried to prevail upon her to let her hair down. She generally only succumbed on special occasions like one of the children's birthdays.

I felt like a tackling dummy. Presently my emotional balance bounced buck. I gritted my teeth and said to myself, "You're damned right, Buster ..... one cripple ...... coming up!"

John's gallbladder problems were to continue to worsen, and within a year or so he was hospitalized to have it removed. He had also developed angina and had at least one heart attack over the next few years, largely putting an end to his ability to get Rainie up and take her out. In addition, being sedentary and without the rigorous PT atmosphere of Warm Springs, Rainie put on considerable weight and lost some muscle tone, making it more difficult for her to withstand the rigors of moving from bed to wheelchair to car and back again.

By about 1959, she almost never left her bed, except for the all-too-frequent trips to the hospital when a cold would compromise her breathing ability. Naturally, the family watched her carefully for any signs of on-coming disease; when the children had a cold, they were directed to enter through the basement door and rush upstairs to their bedrooms to avoid infecting mother.

At the first sign of the sniffles, Rainie would remain sitting up in her home "hospital bed" hunched over a steaming pot of tea, hoping the steam would loosen the mucus and allow her lungs to breathe more freely. When that failed, an ambulance would be called, she would be bundled off to Bergen Pines and placed either in an iron lung or on a rocking bed until the virus ran its course and her breathing ability returned to normal. Over the remaining years of her life, this probably occurred an average of once or twice a year. For years, even after her death, the sound of a siren in the distance would bring back to the author memories of his mother being rushed off for yet another life-saving stay in the hospital.

Daily life in the handicapped "nest"

Rainie's "nest" was a marvel of ingenuity and "high-technology," 1950s- and 1960s-style. She spent her time in a hospital bed, and in those days such beds had few of the amenities one expects during a hospital stay today. Her bed had two sets of hand-cranks, one to raise and lower the upper half of the bed and the other to allow her to raise her knees. Of course, there was no remote control, so someone else would have to adjust her bed for her each time she felt the need to move. She kept a side-rail only on the right side of the bed and, by means of "tricks" learned at Warm Springs, was able to pull herself onto her right side to sleep.

Bed sores are a constant risk for bed-ridden patients, and Rainie was no exception. She was unable to lift herself up and shift her bottom, so someone had to help her adjust her position several times a day. Nevertheless, she developed one permanent bed sore that, by some miracle, never grew large enough or became infected enough to seriously threaten her health or life. To relieve the pressure around the sore, she used a horseshoe-shaped piece of foam rubber, which again, someone had to adjust for her periodically. This situation must have been difficult for her—polio destroys the motor nerves that allow movement, but not the sensory nerves that convey feeling—but she never complained about her immobility.

Rainie, of course, was unable to get up to use the toilet or take a bath. Someone had to put her on and take her off a bed pan several times a day, a chore that occasionally fell to Toby or—even more rarely—to Chris. For the most part, either John or the live-in assistant handled her bathroom needs. Similarly, John or the housekeeper would administer a "bed bath" once or more a week, rolling her over and washing her with a soapy cloth. She was able to brush her own teeth (with a hospital tooth brushing catch basin) and comb her own hair.

Unable to get up from bed, and with her husband no longer able easily to take her out, Rainie was lucky enough to find a doctor, a dentist, and even a hair-dresser who would make occasional house calls and see to her needs.

With a little ingenuity, Rainie became amazingly self-sufficient. Although her Warm Springs dreams of being able to cook and help around the house were never to materialize, she created an arms-length environment in which she had almost every-thing she needed. It started with her lap tray, a wicker tray with deep and wide pockets on each side that held many of her "essentials": cigarettes, lighter, makeup, pencils, pens, writing paper, phone book, back-scratcher, and other assorted items. Next to her bed, on the side where she had more arm mobility, she had a three-tiered table on wheels. She could only reach the top shelf, but

it contained other items she might need, including a small black-and
-white television that she could watch and turn off after everyone
else had gone to bed.

In the early 1960s, a generous neighbor bought her a new,
larger television that actually had a *remote control*. Though a big,
clunky affair, it allowed her to watch a bigger picture and enabled
the children to sit on the couch in her room and watch evening TV
with her. Rainie had a few favorite soap operas, but especially
loved to watch the World Series and the quadrennial political
conventions, equally great sport in her view. There were a few
programs, however, that she refused to watch:

- The popular drama, *Sea Hunt*, starring Lloyd Bridges,
  because she couldn't stand to watch scenes in which
  someone was struggling to breathe underwater or
  reliant on machinery for his oxygen.
- *Beat the Clock*, a popular game show in which
  contestants tried to accomplish zany tasks in less than
  a minute. The effort and energy wasted on such mean-
  ingless undertakings offended her since every necessary chore she undertook required such great effort.

Rainie by no means wasted all her time watching TV,
however. Again, with a little ingenuity she performed an amazing

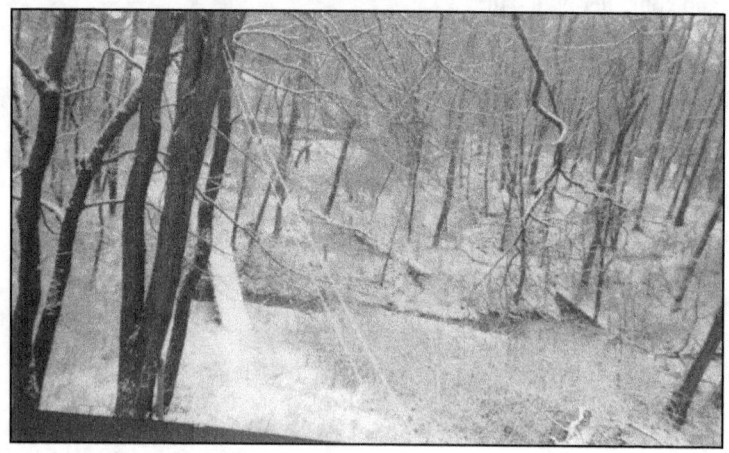

"Clarke's Canyon"
The woods behind the house and view from Rainie's room.

148

array of tasks and pursued both a job and a wide range of hobbies, despite having the use of one arm only from the elbow and the other only from the shoulder. Among the things she enjoyed doing were:

- Sewing. Rainie sewed both by hand and *with a sewing machine.* She had an old Singer model that she would have someone place on her tray. She ran the cord to the pedal around her neck and pressed the "foot" switch with her chin. She was able to thread the needle, change bobbins, and sew a wide variety of items, including clothes for the children (especially for Toby), doll clothes, and craft items, some of which she tried to sell. Sewing was a difficult and sometimes dangerous task, however. One day, after the author had returned from school, Rainie was sewing something when I heard her scream for help. Running into her bedroom, I saw that she had driven the machine needle clear through her fingernail and out the other side of her finger. Very gingerly, I helped her back out the needle and got her a bowl of rubbing alcohol to soak her finger in to prevent infection.

- Typing. John and Rainie had an old manual typewriter (electric typewriters were either not available or were prohibitively expensive at the time). She would have it placed on her tray and spend hours typing poetry, stories, and reports for her job.

- Shopping. Rainie took full advantage of the mail order business. Credit cards were still a thing of the future—a few major stores had introduced an innovation: "charge plates" with which one could charge one's in-store purchases and receive a later bill—but major mail order companies like Sears and Montgomery Wards would allow a person to order "COD" (cash-on-delivery"). When the item arrived, the purchaser would hand over a check to the delivery-man. Rainie would spend hours pouring over the catalogues, looking for just the right clothes for Toby and selecting Christmas and birthday presents for John and the kids.

- Crafts. Always artistic, Rainie had learned a number of crafts at Warm Springs and expanded her repertoire by self-teaching. She made costume jewelry, hand-made greeting cards, and drew and painted. In one of her schemes to make a little "pin money," she arranged for a local wallpaper store to give her old sample books. She would cut the samples to fit boxes of matches, glue them on, then embellish the designs with sequins, beads, and other ornaments.

- <u>Reading and writing</u>. Rainie loved to read—poetry, mystery novels, plays, comedy, history, classics—and had an amazing range of knowledge for someone without a college education. She read plays from Shakespeare and Noel Coward (who was a personal friend). She devoured a multi-volume history of the English Plantagenet dynasty and the humorous accounts of suburban life by Erma Bombeck. Her favorite poets ranged from Ogden Nash to Edna St. Vincent Millay to Robert Frost, along with the sonnets of the Bard. Her notebooks are full of vocabulary lists, classical allusions, French expressions, and possible rhymes.

An active social life

Rainie also carried on an active social life, despite her inability to "go out." One of the staples of her bedside table was her trusty red rotary-dial telephone with which she would keep in touch with neighbors and friends. As a youngster, it seemed that more often than not when I returned from school, mother would have a visitor. Among the most frequent and memorable were:

- Beverly Knecht, a young and attractive gal who lived several blocks away. She was blind, the result of brittle diabetes, and would die before her 40th birthday. She and Rainie loved to sit and chat, exchanging ideas for stories, working on poetry together, or just chatting.
- Ruth (and Dave) Horan, a well -to-do couple who lived on the wealthier end of Mountain

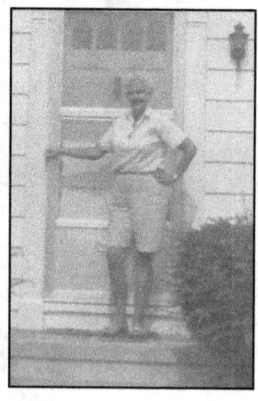

Ruth Horan

150

Avenue and who took the three Clarke children almost every year for a week's vacation at one of the New Jersey shore's swankiest hotels. Ruth donated a good deal of her time to typing books in Braille and would often stop by to chat.

- Celia Selikoff, wife of the eminent Dr. Selikoff, who would often stop by with little gifts, or just to check in on Rainie, often bringing her pair of dachshunds.

- Mary (and Jerry) Mullowney and Lee (and Bill) Donohue, both good Catholic families who seemed to be in competition for who could have more children. (The Mullowneys won by a small margin.) Rainie would occasionally call on them for assistance, especially where expertise with children might be needed. The Donohues would also share their crop of rhubarb every summer, and mother would delight in having a fresh strawberry-rhubarb pie.

- A kind, elderly gentleman, whose name I have forgotten, who lived in an 18th century house—the oldest in the neighborhood—about a block away, who would come by almost every week in the summer with arms full of fresh produce from his garden.

In addition, visitors would sometimes stop by after church on Sunday, occasionally bringing Rainie flower arrangements used during the service.

Although Rainie no longer was able to go out to parties, she and John hosted an annual New Year's Eve affair that was always crowded with old friends and well-wishers. In exchange for being able to stay up extra late to greet the new year, the children were always dragooned into serving as waiters, so long as we would abide by one of Rainie's and John's favorite sayings: "Children should be seen and not heard." During the summers, especially the first few after Rainie's return home, she and John would also occasionally host a "luau" in the backyard, complete with Chinese lanterns festooning the patio, a barbeque pit, and copious mixed drinks for the adults.

The children's birthdays were also the occasion for similar festivities. The two boys, both with birthdays in the month of June, often shared a party, with guests, games, play in the extensive

151

woods behind the house, watermelon (and the injunction that everyone was to spit the seeds over the back hill), and grilled hamburgers and hot dogs. Toby's birthday being in October was often the occasion for a fall party, with corn shocks, Indian corn, a big bonfire, and music.

Raising Cain—and Abel

Rainie had the unenviable task of trying to raise—from bed—two very active and often mischievous boys as well as a much better behaved and helpful little junior mother, Toby.

Even as little boys, Chris and Tim were both inseparable and incompatible. Enjoined to do, or not do, something, Chris would yell and scream defiance, pout and cry with frustrated unhappiness, stamp his feet and mutter imprecations—then go and do what was requested. Tim, on the other hand, was all sweet reasonableness, readily agreeing to whatever was asked, then as soon as he was out of immediate parental grasp would merrily go his way and leave whatever task he had been assigned undone or proceed to do what he had just been enjoined *not* to do.

In several letters to Rainie at Warm Springs, John pretty well caught the dynamic between the boys—a dynamic that persisted until the boys went off to boarding school at around the age of 10.

> [Early February, 1955] Last night was a big deal. Timmy [3½] and Chris [5½] had baths TOGETHER and had a wonderful time. Miraculously (after much persuasion) they DIDN'T mess up the bathroom. I haven't been letting [them] in together because they make such a mess but they PROMISED last nite — AND they lived up to it. Left them in quite a while while I made up my bed (sheets dried outdoors yesterday). Then Timmy GOT TO put on Chris' poodle-doodles [sleeper pajamas] because Chris has outgrown them — and was THAT a big deal?? Really grownup. We all sat in a circle on the floor and talked and had our prayers there and then to bed without ANY trouble. UNUSUAL! This morning Timmy was very proud that he had kept his "big-boy" p.j.'s dry all nite.

[Early March, 1955] Have just sent Chris and Timmy up to the nursery to play. They have been in the basement for about an hour but I don't want them to get too cold. Playing COWBOY. There was a pair of boots with heels in the Newberry box. Don't fit Timmy at all but for awhile they can't hurt his feet too bad. Chris has a pair which someone else gave him a while back. Oh, Timmy is a fiddle playing COWBOY because now, no matter what game he plays, he has to be JACK BENNY, 'cause he likes Rochester so much. Don't ask me to figure it out, that's the reason I always get. Chris changes character hourly and does a pretty good job of keeping his characterizations straight among the Lone Ranger, Tonto, Roy [Rogers], Gene [Autry], and a half dozen other heroes.

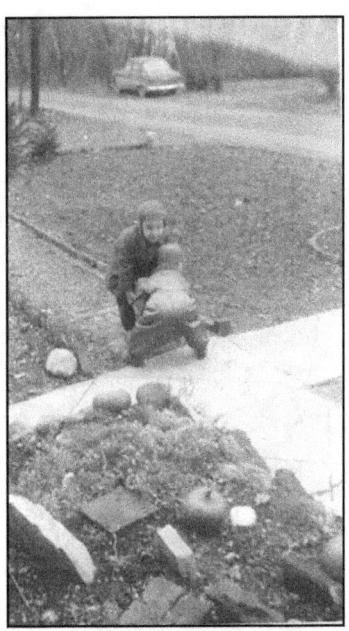

Chris and Timmy struggling to bring in a box of groceries, around 1954.

Half of the day they play together BEAUTIFULLY and I love to sneak up to hear them -- the OTHER half they scream and carry on till I think they will kill each other. Timmy loves to get Chris in all kinds of trouble. He'll tease him, then when Chris takes a poke at him, runs screaming, "Chris hit me in the head - beat me over the back - kicked me" (and a million other things which "Chris" does to him).

The children's antics alternately cause hilarity and humiliation. At dinner one night, Toby was reporting on what she had learned at school that day. "And Paul Bunyon dragged his ax all over the West," she told the family assembled around the table.

153

John almost strangled on his coffee. "He dragged his *what?*," he demanded. Another time, Toby dashed downstairs, interrupting a visit from a deaconess from the church, loudly complaining to Rainie, "Mother! Mother! Chris just called me a bastard!" Timmy, a five or six year-old caught in the basement after someone turned out the lights, hollered, "Who turned out the lights? I can't see a damned thing!" For his part, Chris somewhere had picked up a phrase and some suggestive dance moves and spent several weeks prancing around, shaking his bottom, wagging his finger like Cab Calloway, and repeating "Hot Butt Mambo."

In retrospect, it's embarrassing to admit that we boys saw Rainie's disability as a challenge and invitation to evade parental supervision and get away with anything short of bloody murder. When we were going out, Rainie, of course, always wanted to quiz us on where we were going, what we were going to be doing, how long we would be, and to admonish us to be careful, not to get into trouble... a catechism we assiduously attempted to avoid.

We took advantage of every opportunity to slip our leashes unnoticed. For example, when Rainie was receiving her daily morning bed pan, and the curtains to her room were closed, we would silently sneak down the stairs, stealthily open the front door,

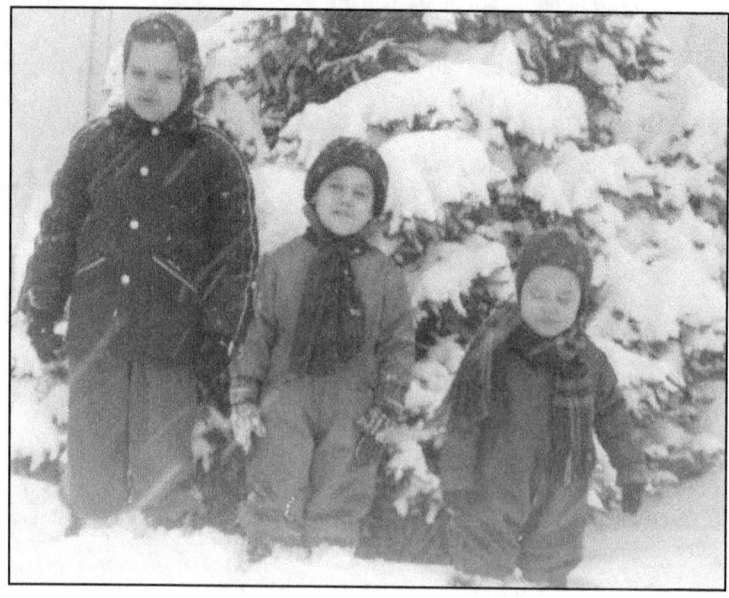

and head out for a day of adventure, ignoring her calls if she should happen to hear us at the door. On one occasion, we demonstrated our own considerable ingenuity in evading supervision. Rainie was suffering from a mild cold, but the doctor had suggested we rent and use a rocking bed and keep her at home rather than take her to the hospital. Over the next week or so, we mastered the art of waiting at the top of the stairs until the bed rocked so far back that mother's vision was blocked by the raised foot of the bed. That was our signal to silently sneak down the stairs. We couldn't make it all the way past her on one cycle of elevation and decline, so we would hide just out of view on the first floor until the bed rocked back again, putting her head below her feet and temporarily blocking her vision. Like Batman and Robin, we would silently dash past her room, through the dining room and kitchen, down the basement stairs and out the back door.

Despite these rare and well-celebrated successes, we were simply no match for Rainie's motherly intuition and wiles. The boys' bedroom on the second floor had a window that opened onto the roof of the sun porch where mother lived. We loved to take out the screen and sneak out onto the roof, usually just for the adventure of it. With a certainty approaching scientific certitude, mother would detect our presence on the roof and, through the "squawk box" that verbally connected the upstairs and her bedside—she would yell at us to get our "little butts" off the "G'dam roof." We were mystified for years how she detected us. We *knew* we were as stealthy as a superhero and as quiet as a cat. We had taken our shoes off, moved only inches at a time, and frozen at the slightest sound. Did she have Superman's X-ray vision? His super-hearing? Was she clairvoyant? How *did* she almost always know we were on the roof. It was only years later that we found out. She wasn't endowed with powers far beyond those of mortal men. Unless it was high noon, she could see our shadows on one side of the sun porch or the other and knew we were up to our old tricks.

Toby, while far less troublesome than the boys, had one great "fault": she loved to read, and would often stay up far past her bedtime engrossed in some novel or other. Somehow mother always knew and, using the infernal squawk box would holler at Toby to turn out the light and go to bed. Again, we all pondered what super-sense she possessed to be able to discern Toby's post-bedtime reading habits. Toby's bedroom was on the back side

155

of the house, across the hall from the boys'. Mother could see out the sun porch window that her light was still on. Even after Toby took a play from our playbook and deviously pulled the covers over her head to read by the dimness of a flashlight, mother would still espy the faint glow through the window and put an abrupt end to the surreptitious late-night escape into the alternate reality of good fiction.

As "normal" children, of course, it almost never occurred to us that we weren't "playing fair." Mother wasn't handicapped; she was just mother. And a child's duty is to test parental limits and see what you can get away with. In retrospect, one can only imagine the frustration and psychological pain of a loving mother who couldn't get up and rush to soothe a crying child, kiss a "boo-boo," tie her children's shoes, dress them for school, give them a bath, make them an after-school snack, tend a son or daughter with a fever or cold, take them shopping or on an outing, or swat a naughty bottom.

This frustration must have been only partially offset by our nightly ritual of climbing up on her bed—sometimes singly, sometimes all at once, sometimes with one or more dogs—to give her hugs and kisses all in a wiggling tangle and say goodnight. As we got older, we would sometimes do our homework in her room, asking for her help, or watch evening TV with her. On occasion, we would rub her feet—a distasteful task, given their dryness and lifeless feel, but one we did to show affection in partial compensation for our transgressions. But her inability to do for her children the manifold tasks that "normal" mothers of the time did must have been a hidden pain that we scarcely noticed or recognized.

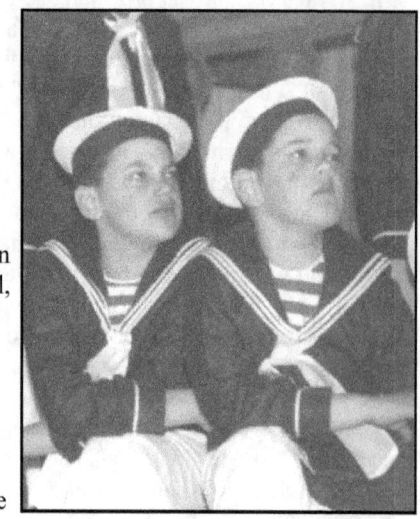

Chris (left) and Tim (right) in Gilbert and Sullivan's *Pirates of Penzance*, while at St. Thomas Church Choir School about 1962.

At age 10, Chris was admitted to St. Thomas Church Choir School in New York City, one of the few full-time boarding choir schools in the country. Two years later, Tim joined him there. All things considered, it was a rational—maybe even good—decision, given the chaotic environment at home, the burdens on John and Rainie, and the scholarships, excellent education, and cultural opportunities the school offered. But it was no "Goodbye, Mr. Chips" experience, and the boys were anything but happy. The school ran from 5th to 8th grade, after which Chris returned to the Ridgewood public school system; two years later, Tim matriculated at the Hinkley school, a preparatory school in Maine. Toby, meanwhile, stayed at home, attending junior high and high school in Ridgewood.

Time passed. Summers were filled with play in the woods, long-distance bicycle rides, hours at Ridgewood's wonderful man-made lake/swimming pool—and book reports, penmanship practice under the watchful eye of Mother, and for Chris and Toby, part-time jobs and/or advanced classes in high school.

From penury to (Relative) Security

The Clarke finances remained precarious after Rainie returned home. John was able only to pick up occasional part-time or relief work, the income from which was barely able to keep the wolf from the door. John picked up a steady Saturday job for a while and briefly even worked at selling used cars; friendly well-wishers recommended a change of career: "How about working as a nursery man? You obviously have a green thumb," one suggested. "You could land a job as a restaurant cashier," another opined. Mrs. Newberry apparently even offered John a job with the new, huge store their family was planning to open, and one "friend" suggested, "Why doesn't Toby peddle your [Rainie's] gadgets after school? Nobody can resist a child."

Finances were so tight—although the children never realized it—that by November 1955, two years after Rainie was stricken with polio, the Village of Ridgewood entered in the local newspaper a "Notice of Sale of Property for Non-Payment of Taxes" on John and Rainie's house and property for the grand sum of $4.60 in unpaid taxes for 1953 and 1954. Somehow, John scraped together the less-than-five-dollars to stave off foreclosure.

The family poverty, as was usual with the Clarkes, provided not only moments of worry, anguish, and embarrassment, but rare moments of gallows humor. Around Thanksgiving of 1955, after Rainie had returned home, Mrs. Newberry delivered a load of canned food which included *eleven* large cans of pumpkin. John made a fresh pumpkin pie every day for a week (one reason, no doubt, that more than 50 years later, the author shies away from this autumn "delicacy" as if it were rat poison), and used all his imagination and country upbringing to think of every creative way possible to utilize canned pumpkin to feed the family. A few days later, another well-meaning family friend proudly arrived at the door bearing—a fresh pumpkin pie! Poor Toby nearly mortally insulted the charitable lady by moaning to her mother, "Oh, Mom, not *another pie!"*

In another "humorous" twist, Toby proudly and cheerfully helped her second grade class prepare food baskets for "poor people"—on the same day Social Services called to ask if we could use one.

The holidays bring out the best in most of us, and the festive season of 1955 was no exception. Shortly before Thanksgiving, food starting pouring into the Clarke house as if someone had turned the cornucopia upside down on our doorstep. The unexpected and much appreciated windfall had its comedic side as well, however. John was kept busy racing up and down the stairs between basement freezer—bought in the salad days immediately after the family moved into the house—and the front door, hiding each load of food as it arrived so as not to embarrass the donors or make them feel their contributions were unwelcome or unnecessary. By the end of the day before Thanksgiving, John had stowed away some 65 pounds of turkey and assorted other comestibles, enough to feed a small brigade, never mind a needy family of five. As it was, the family ended up getting Rainie dressed, in her wheelchair, in and out of the car, and into the house of Dave and Ruth Horan— quite a safari for a move of less than a block up the street—to be their guests for Thanksgiving dinner.

Christmas that year was memorable as well, the first one in three years with Rainie home and presiding. She had done her best to squeeze the few dollars the family could afford into a handful of mail-order presents for the kids and the traditional bottle of Vitalis hair tonic and new T-shirts for John. But neighbors, friends, and charity groups all pitched in to assure a Christmas tree piled high with gifts, especially for the kids, and apparently quite a few donations to help the Clarkes get by financially.

No doubt, despite the realization that they were the objects of charity (see next page), John and Rainie must have delighted in seeing the joy of their youngsters—now nine, six, and four, the perfect ages for the magic of Christmas—squealing in delight and running around playing with their new toys or trying on their new clothes. The holiday spirit was to be relatively short-lived, however, as shortly after Christmas, Rainie had to be rushed back to Bergen Pines with a cold for the second time since her return home.

The next year (1956) was another hand-to-mouth period, full of parental attempts to earn enough to get by while fooling the children into believing that life was normal and everything was fine. John continued his Saturday job, leaving nine-year-old Toby to run the house for the day. Rainie picked up some work, doing a television survey for the PTA on proper shows for children to be allowed to watch—all the while listening distantly to Chris and Tim upstairs watching on a donated TV such programs as *Dragnet* and the movie, *King Kong*. If only the blue-stockings of the PTA had known!

Easter came, and soft-hearted, well-meaning Daddy brought home a basket full of little ducklings. "Well," he told Rainie, "after they grow a little, we can let them swim in the pond down the hill." Mother's "Maraduke" seemed to get into everything, but would cuddle warmly with her on her bed. The little ducks (predictably) would never stay where they were supposed to, and John indelibly imprinted upon the boys' minds the sight of an adult man wielding a six foot bamboo pole, standing up to his thighs in a muddy and mucky pond, swatting at their precious ducklings, yelling "Get out of that filthy water, you little bastards!"

Timmy broke down and retorted to his father, "Donald is not a bastard!," undoubtedly having no idea what the word even meant. In any event, it wasn't long before the ducks grew up, wised, up, and lifted up on grown-up wings to disappear over the

"Charity"

[Rainie Clarke's unfinished and unpublished autobiography, which has served as a major source for much of this book, was titled *Charity Begins at Home*. She chose to begin it with a quote from I Corinthians, 13:13: "And now abideth faith, hope, and charity, these three; but the greatest of these *is* charity." Her feelings about the meaning of "charity" are pretty clearly expressed in the following paragraphs, which she had intended to include somewhere in the chapters of her autobiography on the years immediately after her return from Warm Springs, the most difficult financial times in the Clarke family.]

Charity is a word which has suffered tremendously by mis-usage. In it's original context, it meant love and a brotherly concern for one's fellow man. To a few people it still holds such a connotation. Today, unfortunately, the word, to a vast majority of people, implies "a hand-out to assuage one's social conscience." Charity, given with love and empathy is a great spiritual experience for giver and receiver alike. Charity extended with sympathy and embarrassment may act as a spiritual cathartic for the donor, but it misses the point entirely if it humiliates (as distinguished from humbles) the recipient. John tells a story from his childhood which illustrates this statement.

In the small town in Ohio where his Aunt Maud lived, it was the custom of the ladies of her church to prepare a Thanksgiving dinner for the unfortunate and under-privileged members of the community. It was served at the town hall on Thanksgiving night. Aunt Maud contributed food, time and a considerable talent for cooking, working industriously for several days to assure the success of the occasion. But she spoiled the effect of her offering when, after every Thanksgiving at home, she would arise and announce to the assembled family, "Come on. Let's all go down town and watch the poor people eat." She failed to distinguish the dividing line between charity and self-righteousness.

horizon for less volatile and hopefully more companionable climes.

Spring came, and with it another cold, and another trip to Bergen Pines for Rainie. Shortly thereafter, the children came down with Chicken Pox, putting the fear of God into John and Rainie about what might be the impact if she were to catch *that* on top of all her other problems.

Out of poverty — at last

Late 1956 and 1957, at long last, brought lasting good news. Rainie, surprisingly, was the first to "find work." In December 1956, she was hired by the National Broadcasting Company (NBC) as a paid "radio monitor."

The lesser part of the job consisted of tracking NBC programs, especially its "soap operas," and commenting on such issues as acting quality, plot lines, and the like. The majority of her time was to be spent, however, monitoring the competition (ABC and CBS) to inform her NBC bosses what other radio stations were doing well or badly. Rainie set up her own business, called "Filtered Tips," to provide this service, and was contracted at the princely sum of $50.00 a week, a virtual windfall for a family used to limping by on uneven and sporadic income. She continued this work until March 1961.

After years of part-time, temporary, seasonal, and pick-up work, John finally landed in the Big Time. He was hired on as a permanent staff announcer at NBC in New York in June, 1957. After more than 30 years in "the business," and well over a decade in the New York area, he had made it to the top. There was no more prestigious job at the time in broadcasting than being a permanent announcer for NBC, the leading network. In addition to a regular schedule on WNBC radio and a good salary, John was able to supplement his income by doing commercial announcements and station breaks on NBC-TV, as well as whatever freelance work he could find and wanted to do. (He retired from NBC after more than 20 years and died in 1981.)

Filtered Tips

Rainie used her position as a consultant to NBC to pitch a number of ideas for programs, suggest "jingles" (short, catchy commercial phrases or tunes to entice listeners to tune into certain programs), and to hone her writing craft. A number of her reports to her boss, Jerry Danzig, included cover notes that are both poetic and highly amusing:

(February 27, 1958) Dear Jerry,

Little drops of water,
little grains of sand,
make a mighty ocean,
and a blister on your heel!

Such is the outlook on a dreary day. Ah, *printemps!* As a matter of fact, ANY *temps* but these *temps!*

Best wishes, Rainie.

In August 1957, after having monitored and criticized for some time the NBC program "The Affairs of Doctor Gentry," Rainie sent her boss the following note:

Cheri Jerry,

An addendum to the report: some good fairy must have attended your birth, because you were most certainly blessed with the divine gift of patience. And it is precisely that gift of patience to which "The Affairs of Doctor Gentry" owes much of its success. Nor should the writer's willingness to listen to suggestions and to work hard be underestimated. He has spun gold out of straw through sheer diligence. But how fortunate for the show, and for NBC that you had the patience to wait for the miracle! "Gentry" is now one lulu of a show.

Kindest wishes.

Sincerely, la dame sans merci.

Demonstrating how she could be both highly critical, yet amusing and charming in delivering bad news, Rainie wrote Jerry Danzig in September 1957 about a program, "Pepper Young's Family," that was not doing well.

162

Dear Jerry, Prince of Good Fellows:

Although there is every possibility that after you have read my report, you may not feel like a prince of good fellows. Instead, you may sit there at your work bench, fingering your pearl-handled letter opener, and ponder just which area of my swan-like neck would make the best point of insertion. I should have no kick coming, seeing as how I have stuck it out.

With apologies to Omar and Friends

The moving finger writes and having writ
moves on; nor all my piety nor wit
assisted me in being discreet.
"Pepper" is still a crock of —- shredded wheat!

Yourn, Rainie

Facing yet another upheaval over a hiatus in domestic help, and therefore a tardy report to her boss, on April 12, 1958, Rainie wrote:

Dear Jerry,

Dust is dusting
Buds are busting
Paint is moulting
Maids are bolting
The whole development's revolting!

I just *ain't* a domesticated fowl.

Your adult delinquent,
Rainie

Showing both her wit and erudition, on September 23, 1958 Rainie wrote to Jerry Danzig:

'Tis the transplanting
season and our front yard

163

looks like Birnum Woods.
Ah, well. We'll just rename
the place "Dunsinane".

Best wishes to all, Rainie

Living through another un-air-conditioned summer in hot
and humid Ridgewood, Rainie wrote her boss on July 14, 1958:

Dear Jerry,

The days of the dog,
July and Aug.
slip by in a shroud of
humid smog.
But I'll bet by far
that by Feb. and Mar.
we'll whistle for things
the way they are.

The dual employment finally put the family in the position
to look for full-time, live-in help to keep house and take care of
Rainie's needs while John worked and the kids went to school.

The Hired Help's Revolving Door

Rainie's inability to do routine household chores—and
John's sometimes erratic and mostly all-night work schedule—
meant the family required live-in help. Upon Rainie's return from
Warm Springs, the National Foundation for Infantile Paralysis had
arranged for a two-week stay by a helper whom Rainie named
"Meadows" in her unpublished autobiography. Rainie described the
family's first experience with what would prove to be a long line of
diverse and interesting "helpers," some of whom stayed one night
(and one only half an hour) before deciding the job was too difficult
or distasteful. Some stayed for months and a few lasted longer than
that, resulting in our later estimate of having had something like 60
live-in housekeepers over the roughly nine years after Rainie
returned from Warm Springs.

"Meadows"
By
Rainie Clarke

[Upon arriving at the airport, returning from Warm Springs.]

"Where are the children?" I asked. "They're in the building with Meadows, looking at the gift shop." John said.[1]

"Who's Meadows?"

"The housekeeper."

"Then you were able to get one. That's a relief."

"Well, yes and no. Don't get too attached to her. She can only stay for two weeks."

"Oh? How did you happen to get her? Did you find her yourself?'"

"No."

"The county Chapter?"

John answered, "No. They said finding a housekeeper was against their policy."

"Well, how ?"

"National Foundation sent her out from New York. She specializes in taking patients home and getting them organized."

"What's she like?"

"You'll see in a minute. I think you'll like her. The children do."

---

[1] I suppose there's no harm so many years later in revealing that Meadows'" actual name was Dora Barnes, a lovely lady from Barbados.

By this time we had reached the middle of the waiting room and rolled to a stop. Across the room I saw, coming toward me, a charming-looking middle aged woman in a stiffly starched white uniform, ushering three children.

"Darling, this is Willa Meadows. The children call her 'Meadows' and she says she likes it."

I acknowledged Meadows gratefully. It was such a relief to know that someone was going to help us ease into what my recent confreres termed the "adjustment period". I said, "Meadows, it's so good to have you with us."

"Darling little Mrs. Clarke, I am so happy to be here," she replied. I detected the soft cadences of a West Indian accent. I beamed at her. In my whole life nobody had ever called me darling *little* anything. Meadows had made a solid hit !...

Breaking away from a long tenure of hospitalization is a rupture of great psychological proportions. My first two weeks home were cushioned by the capable Meadows. However, as the days went by and I got to know her better I began to realize that, on a long range basis, she was not the ideal person for the job.

Meadows was an uncomplicated personality. She believed in beer and the Brooklyn Dodgers. She did not believe in God.

The beer was not a financial burden as she provided it herself. I could fend off the Brooklyn Dodger broadcasts with the counter-irritant of listening to the New York Giants; but it required more diplomacy than I am ordinarily capable of to control her pointedly atheistic remarks in front of the children.

She was an excellent cook, but heavy handed on the groceries, always making two items do the work of one (a habit which, in our experience, seems to be peculiar to domestic help.) This was a source of irritation to John's Pennsylvania Dutch thrift.

He felt, too, that she was spoiling me. He knew that if I

expected to return to a normal world, I had to learn to accept life on normal terms; that I could not afford the moral degeneration of having every whim satisfied simply because I had experienced unfortunate and limiting physical circumstances. It seemed like a brutal attitude at the time, but I can see now that he was right.

One afternoon Meadows was rummaging through the kitchen cabinets and came across a long unused bottle of rum. She trotted into the living room with it. "Mr. Clarke," she asked, "do you have any Falernum?"

"Falernum?. . .Oh, sure. We keep it in the pantry with the peacock eggs and the evaporated squid juice! What the hell is Falernum?"

"It's a liquor that's made in my home in Barbados. It goes wonderfully with rum."

"I've always wondered what they did in Barbados."

Meadows persisted, "I'm serious, Mr. Clarke. I'd like to buy some Falernum. I am also out of beer. Will you please drive me to a liquor store?"

John sighed and reached for the car keys. He recognizes an impasse when he meets one.

Marble Hill [Ridgewood] is a self-sufficient village. It boasts a buying public of excellent incomes and divergent enough tastes to require an unusually ample selection of delicacies. But it looked like Meadows had Marble Hill stumped. As they pulled up in front of liquor store #6 John said, "Meadows, if they don't have it here, you'll have to settle for Coke. I'm not going all the way to Barbados to get it."

Meadows was right. It is a delicious drink; one part Falernum, one part rum, lemons and limes, served in a large mug over plenty of ice cubes. It is also very rough on the calories.

"Meadows"—Dora Barnes—was to be only the first of a steady stream of characters who would parade through our lives in a colorful and sometime strange circus. With a few memorable exceptions, the vast majority were young, African-American girls recruited from the Deep South by agencies that provided Northern families with domestic help and assured the girls they could make their fortune, escape their mostly rural poverty, and find a nice young man to marry and take care of them. Some had worked hard at home, but few had any idea what they were facing when they entered the Clarke house.

The housekeepers' duties included cleaning, cooking, seeing after the children, and most of all, attending to Rainie's needs. This included providing bed pans several times a day—an unpleasant task in the best of circumstances—giving Rainie bed baths and changing her bed linen at least once a week, and fetching various and sundry articles, including seemingly endless pots of tea, at her request. John had divided off the one large bedroom upstairs to make a small garret, barely wide enough for a single bed, a dresser, and a chair, that was to be the housekeeper's room. She would, of course, share the single bathroom with the rest of the family, including three sloppy and unruly children. She was on duty from early morning (generally around 7:00 am) until late evening (around 9:00 pm), though not continuously employed throughout the day. She was expected to work 5½ days a week, with Sunday and Tuesday evening off. And for this, she was paid the princely sum of $35 dollars a week (the prevailing wage for live-in house-keepers), plus free room and board.

Little wonder few could withstand the rigors of the job for very long. Quite a number, after a few weeks on the job, would take off on Sunday or for their Tuesday evening, head to Patterson, the nearest big city, and never be heard from again. This would leave the family in the lurch for several days until the hiring agency could supply someone new. That meant that John—generally backed up by Toby, then not even a teenager—would have to attend to cooking and Rainie's needs until a new person arrived.

Some of the more memorable characters to pass through the Clarke family circus were:

- The very short-term gal who, after only a few days on the job, waited until the family was all in the backyard for a summer picnic, then cleaned out John's wallet, called a cab, and disappeared.

- *Minnie*, whose parents must have had a great sense of humor or no foresight whatsoever when they named her. Not only did she not look or sound a bit like Minnie Mouse, she was no "mini." Probably about 250 pounds of fluff, Minnie had a backside that we boys cruelly, but secretly, called a "shelf butt." Her fundament stood out so prominently that we swore you could stand a glass of Coke on it. When attending to Rainie, poor Minnie had to lift up her frontal adipose and place it on the edge of the bed, sliding up and down the bed to attend to Rainie's needs. The work soon proved too much for her.

- A couple—the only pair the family ever engaged—named *Beatrice and Jesse*. It was an experiment gone awry in the forlorn hope that two sets of hands would be better than one. Beatrice, so the idea went, could attend to the domestic chores and Rainie's needs, which she did competently, while Jesse could serve as a handyman around the house. Unfortunately, he was most handy at avoiding work while imbibing his favorite brand of *aqua vitae*. In short, he was drunk much of the time. The boys, of course, loved him because he taught us how to whittle, played little games, and let us "help" him with his chores. The final straw was when John assigned him to repaint the boys' bunk beds, providing him with a gallon of bright red enamel paint. When Chris and Tim returned from the garage after having a wonderful time "helping" paint the beds, we were covered in enamel paint, from hair to shoes.

- "The Rhine maiden," as Rainie dubbed her, a stern German *hausfrau* direct from central casting after not making the cut for *Die Valkyrie*. She lasted two weeks, discovered she was allergic to work, and "copped a swan," as Rainie put it.

- Lena, a middle-aged Italian immigrant from the Piedmont who had nothing but scorn and wrath for our next door neighbors, an Italian-American family in which the father was a police officer retired on disability after a motorcycle accident and which contained a first-generation grandfather. She insisted on deprecating the family as *Siciliani*, as if to be of Sicilian ancestry placed them beneath contempt. In her short stay with us, Chris attempted to learn Italian from her, but retained only a few curse words and the useful phrase, "*Bambini essere viduti ma non sentiti*", or "children should be seen but not heard." Somehow, Lena had received a driver's license; asked to drive to Patterson to pick up John after his gallbladder surgery, John swore she nearly gave him a myocardial infarction on the way home with her erratic skills behind the wheel, and almost landed him back in the hospital.

- The young, pretty, almond-skinned African-American girl who proved to be as pleasant as she was competent and hard working. Unfortunately, she was college bound and could only stay the summer. We kids loved her, and John and Rainie probably would have offered to adopt her if only she would stay permanently.
- Peaceful Lillio, as sweet and loving an old lady as her name sounds. We never learned her real age, but rumor had it she was three weeks older than God. She was a devotee of the famous and controversial Philadelphia preacher, Father Divine.[2] Peaceful did her best to convert the family into believers and even took us to one of the movement's potluck suppers, a racially

---

[2] Father Divine (c. 1876 – September 10, 1965), also known as Reverend M.J. Divine, was an African American spiritual leader from about 1907 until his death. His full self-given name was Reverend Major Jealous Divine, and he was also known as "the Messenger" early in his life. He founded the International Peace Mission movement, formulated its doctrine, and oversaw its growth from a small and predominantly black congregation into a multiracial and international church.

Controversially, Father Divine claimed to be God. Some contemporary critics also claimed he was a charlatan, and some suppose him to be one of the first modern cult leaders. However, Father Divine made numerous contributions toward his followers' economic independence and racial equality. For more information, see http://en.wikipedia.org/wiki/Father_Divine.

integrated affair long before racial integration had become commonplace. Peaceful could often be heard in the evenings quietly singing hymns while washing the dishes and talking to Father Divine, asking for his help in getting through the day: "Father," she would say, "I just don't know if I can do it anymore. The work is so hard, but the family needs me. Give me strength." Finally, Peaceful's strength gave out and she decided she had to leave. As a going-away present, the family gave her one of the just-weaned cocker spaniel puppies. "But I don't have anything to carry him in," she sighed. Ever resourceful, John went into the attic and retrieved an old birdcage, just large enough for the puppy to fit into comfortably to accompany Peaceful on her bus journey to Philadelphia. "If anyone gives you a hard time," John told her, "just tell them he's a bird dog."

- Beatrice Prayer, another devoutly religious woman from a fringe group, who finally gave up and quit after trying to covert the "heathen" Clarkes or convince John and Rainie to forgo the "sinful" habit of smoking or the occasional glass of sherry.

Exit Stage Left

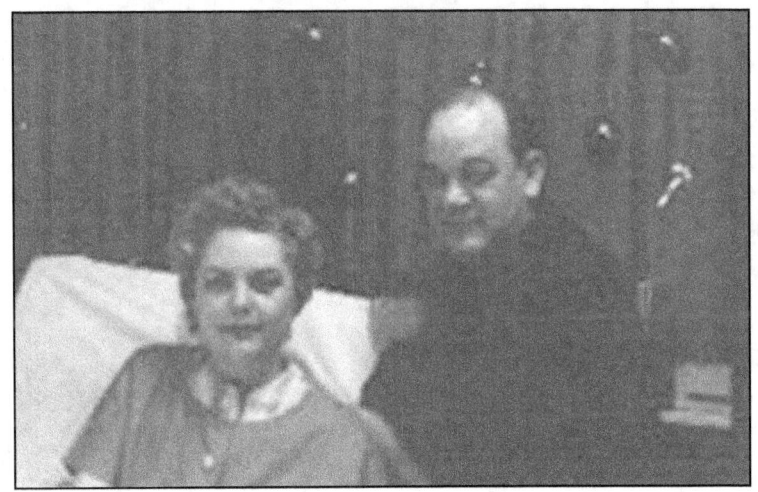

Previous page: One of the last photos of Rainie ever taken and one of the few photos from the 1960s with John and Rainie together. This was likely taken around Christmas 1964. Unfortunately, the quality of the original photo is not very high.

Over the years, John's health continued to deteriorate, with a series of heart attacks and angina that required carrying nitroglycerin at all times. John hosted his all-night radio program, with an added regular routine of daytime and evening television station breaks and commercials that sometimes necessitated staying in New York over night. Rainie continued her productive efforts, but the marriage had slowly cooled, no doubt the result of spending less and less time together, John's long-sublimated frustrations with the situation, constant financial worries, the strains of raising children and the constant turnover of household help, and John's increasingly heavy drinking. By the early 1960s, while Chris and Tim were away at boarding school, the home was becoming an unhappy place, full of tension.

By late-June of 1965, Toby had been home about a week from college—her freshman year at Ohio Wesleyan University, where she had immersed herself in the study of English literature and long Russian novels and attempted to find a sense of security after many years of family tension, responsibility beyond her years, and the usual angst of late adolescence. Tim had returned from Hinkley, and Chris was awaiting the start of a high school summer school class in U.S. history that he was taking for extra credit.

The years of stress had finally caught up with John in June 1965, and Rainie received a call that John had been admitted to the hospital in New York after suffering a heart attack at work. He was also thought to be suffering from exhaustion and something of a "nervous breakdown," complicated by his lifelong smoking habit, and his excessive drinking. These were the days long before routine angioplasty, stents, or cardiac bypass surgery. We were informed that he would likely be there for several weeks of rest, rehabilitation, and efforts to break his unhealthy habits. Though worried, the family took the news in stride. After all, Dad had been in the hospital before and always returned O.K.

But, as had so often happened with the Clarke family, trouble never entered the home unaccompanied. Within a few days, Rainie came down with a cold. The children attempted to nurse her at home, providing endless pots of steaming tea and sitting up with her throughout the night as she struggled to breath and fight off the virus. But, as had also happened so many times before, home care proved not to be enough and Rainie was rushed back to Bergen

175

Pines with Toby riding in the ambulance. Her boyfriend later brought her back home. After almost 10 years since her first admittance, and nearly as much time since polio had been eradicated by the Salk, and then Sabin, vaccines, the young medical staff was totally inexperienced in dealing with a seriously ill polio patient. Rainie was put on a rocking bed, with orders to the nurses to watch her closely for any deterioration.[1]

Toby—at 18, the only one with a driver's license—served as chauffeur; all three of us visited her the evening after her admittance, and she seemed in good spirits and in good hands. The next evening, a Saturday, Toby and Tim stopped by to see her, but for some reason, Chris stayed home, a decision he would regret for years. By late evening, Toby (18), Chris (having turned 16 only a day earlier), and Tim (14 on June 1) were at home and asleep.

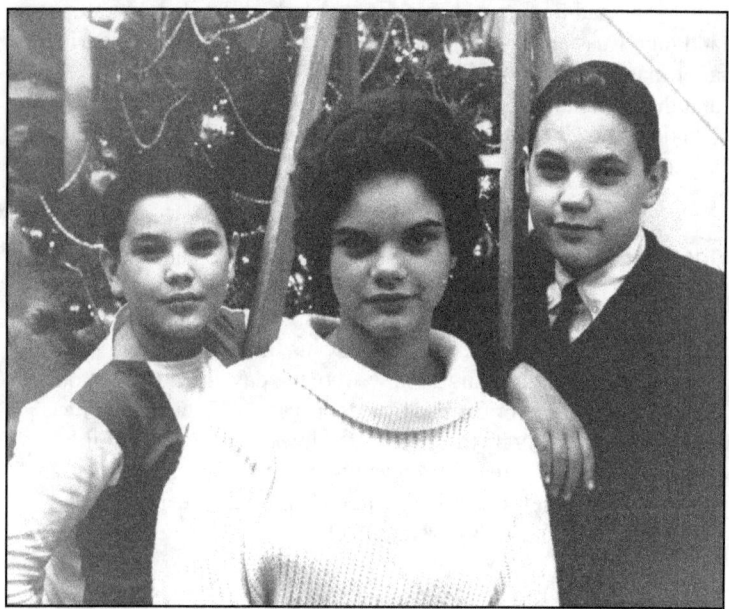

Tim (left), October ("Toby", center) and Chris (right) about 1964.

---

[1] Some 50 years later, the only remaining survivors—Toby and Chris—cannot remember whether John was informed that Rainie had been hospitalized. If so, every effort would have been made to minimize his stress by making her condition seem "routine" and non-life-threatening.

                                *   *   *

Sunday morning, June 25, 1965, a few minutes before 7:00
am: All three Clarke children were sound asleep, looking forward
to sleeping in before going back to Bergen Pines to see Mother
again. The ringing phone jolted us all awake. Blearily, Toby
answered it. "Hello…"

"Is this the Clarke residence?," said a heavily accented
South Asian voice on the other end of the line.

"Yes. Who's calling?"

"This is Dr. Khan (or Subramanian or Singh or whatever;
in her sleepy condition, Toby hardly understood the speaker.) "I am
berry sahree to inform you that Mrs. Clarke expired this morning."

"What? What do you mean 'expired'?," asked the still
sleepy Toby.

"She has passed away. Died," said the disembodied voice
on the other end of the phone.

By now the boys, in the next room, were sitting up in bed
trying to understand the one-sided conversation. Suddenly, Toby
appeared in the doorway, crying. "Boys," she said, "that was the
hospital. The doctor says Mom died overnight of pneumonia."

We all sat in stunned silence as the news penetrated our
sleepy brains. "Died?", we thought. "How can that be? Toby and
Tim just saw her last night and she seemed to be getting better.
She's been to the hospital with a cold a dozen time over the years
and always recovered to return home. Mom? Gone? What the hell
are we supposed to do now?"

                                *   *   *

As usual, Toby rose to the occasion. We all quickly
dressed and she began to make phone calls. One of the first was to
Dad's hospital. We didn't dare call him and tell him ourselves; he
was being treated for a heart attack and we worried that such a call
could push him right over the edge, maybe bringing on a fatal
attack. Toby talked to the nurse on his floor, who quickly contacted

                                177

the doctor. Once they had the story straight, the medical professionals took over.

The doctor appeared at Dad's door. He said, "John, come take a walk with me. Let's go down to the patient lounge at the end of the hall." Arriving there, the doctor handed Dad a cigarette—something he'd been forbidden since he was admitted to the hospital—and said, "You'd better sit down. I have some bad news. Your wife has passed away." Understandably, John was momentarily speechless, then in denial, then he fell apart. The doctor said, "I'm sorry. It's a helluva a blow at a time like this," and told the nurse to give him a heavy sedative and put him back to bed. We called Dad later that day, but the conversation wasn't very coherent.

* * *

Tim and Toby stayed up all night Sunday talking, while Chris, exhausted, went to bed. They found this a strong bonding experience after some five years of limited contact (with Tim away at boarding school and Toby now off in college). Early the next morning we went to a local diner for breakfast to discuss what to do next. John had already visited a local funeral home, discussing possible future arrangements for *himself*, never dreaming that Rainie might die first. We decided that Toby, with Chris playing second fiddle, would visit the funeral home and make the necessary arrangements, while Tim would stay at home. Dad, still hospitalized under heavy sedation was clearly in no shape to make arrangements from his bed in New York.

It must have been quite a sight for an 18-year-old and a barely-16-year-old to enter the funeral home and ask to speak to the funeral director about a funeral. We were greeted by a rather unctuous elderly fellow who proceeded to walk us through the process. We told him the name of the deceased and where her body could be picked up, and he set about retrieving Mom's remains. Then he sat down to fill out a form for submitting an obituary to the local papers.

"O.K., what was your mother's name?," he asked.

"Rainie Clarke," Chris piped up, assuming the position of "man of the house."

"Well, actually," Toby corrected, "Her full and proper name was Lorraine Reynolds Woodruff Clarke."

"When was she born?"

"November 28," Chris replied.

"What year?"

Chris looked at Toby, completely stumped. How old was Mom? He wasn't sure.

"1920," Toby replied.

"Where was she born?," the funeral director asked.

"Florida, I think," said Chris, remembering where Granddad lived.

"No," interjected Toby, "Fort Worth, Texas." "Oh, right," Chris thought, "While Grandpa and Grandma were on the Vaudeville circuit."

"And was this a short or long illness?"

"Short," Chris said, thinking of the few days' hospitalization with the cold.

"Long," Toby replied almost simultaneously, referring to her nearly 10 years with polio.

Chris decided to shut up and let Toby handle the details.

Those details included finding a recent photo of mother so the cosmetologist and hair dresser could make mother look as natural as possible. We drove home and brought one back.

"And how would she want to be dressed?," he asked.

"Well," Chris and Toby whispered to each other, "we certainly can't put her in a casket dressed in the usual smock and pajama bottoms" she wore routinely. The funeral director showed

179

us some perfectly awful Victorian-era lacy shrouds, which we knew would have made Mom turn over in her coffin if we had dressed her in them.

"I'll check at home and find an appropriate outfit," Toby assured.

*   *   *

The two left, uncertain whether to laugh or cry. This was crazy. A couple of teenagers in charge of a funeral. Neither had ever even *been* to one before, and here we were, in charge of making arrangements that (we hoped) Dad would be able to attend and would approve of, and that wouldn't embarrass the family in front of neighbors or John and Rainie's numerous professional colleagues from show business, where everything was done with the precision of military close-order drill and the attention to detail of a presidential State banquet.

"I know one thing," Toby said to Chris as they drove home. "Mom would want to be wearing high heels," something she had loved before being stricken with polio and had, of course, been unable to wear since.

With no suitable clothes at home, Toby set off in the car to buy an appropriate dress or suit, preferably of Mother's favorite color, purple or lavender. She scoured several of the major up-scale department stores in the malls on the road to New York. At store after store, she could find nothing appropriate, later joking with typical Clarke gallows humor that she had thought about asking the sales ladies, "Do you have anything nice in a size 42 for a corpse?"

Finally, as the day began to get late, an increasingly dispirited and weary Toby found a lovely light-blue outfit that would be just right. Now for the high heels. What to do? Luckily, one of Mother's friends came through. Lola Bowden, whose teenaged daughter, "Bets," had baby sat for the three kids during the summers, said she had a pair of nice black three-inch heels that she was willing to give us. Toby dropped off the clothes and shoes at the funeral home. We all went home, showered, dressed, and prepared for the viewing that evening.

When we arrived early that evening, the funeral director asked us to look at Mom's remains and make sure her hair and makeup were acceptable. The hair wasn't quite right, so brave Toby—wanting to make everything perfect for the funeral the next day, when Dad might be able to come—took comb and brush in hand, and touching her first dead body, proceeded to arrange Mom's hair just the way she would have wanted it. With an eye to making Mom look just like Dad would want to remember her, she also insisted that the funeral director replace the pale pink lipstick with a bright red one, the kind Mother had always favored.

* * *

The evening viewing seemed to go by without a hitch, though it remains a blur. Chris and Toby did their best to greet the visitors as adults and accept their condolences in a manner we hoped would make our parents proud. Tim, shell-shocked and too young to deal with death, spent the evening in the waiting room. Somehow, the evening eventually came to an end and we headed home.

The funeral the next day, however, was unforgettable. Toby had called and arranged for flowers and picked the music, including several of Mother's favorites, including "Try to Remember" and "The September Song":

> "Oh, it's a long, long while from May to December
> But the days grow short when you reach September
> When the autumn weather turns the leaves to flame
> One hasn't got time for the waiting game
>
> Oh, the days dwindle down to a precious few
> September, November
> And these few precious days I'll spend with you
> These precious days I'll spend with you."

John had been released for a few hours by his doctor. He was heavily sedated. His and Rainie's longtime boss from NBC, Jerry Danzig, picked him up at the hospital in a limousine and they drove the 25 or so miles to the funeral home. The place was packed—neighbors, friends, church members, doctors, some of their rich and famous acquaintances and friends from show business, and a considerable cohort of co-workers from NBC. When John arrived, we children all broke into tears and ran to hug him.

He went over to see Rainie for a last time—and completely fell apart. Sedated, grieving, and in shock from the suddenness of her departure, he bawled, with nose running and tears streaming down his face. Chris pulled out a handkerchief to wipe off his face, trying to keep Dad from being embarrassing in front of all his friends. John bent over and kissed Rainie on the forehead, then took Chris by the hand and insisted he touch his mother to say goodbye. This was the first time I had ever seen a dead body and I was extremely reluctant to touch her. He insisted, and I was shocked and repulsed to find her so cold. Poor Tim, only 14, wouldn't even come out of the waiting room to see his mom in her coffin and didn't join the service until they had closed the casket.

Somehow, we got through the service, the long line of well wishers and condolence givers, and got Dad back in the limousine to head back to New York and his hospital bed.

After it was all over, the three kids piled in Toby's car and, with the hangman's humor that had seen us through so many difficult times, went out to lunch where we laughed, and cried, and remembered all the wonderful times we had enjoyed with the talented, funny, optimistic, supportive, and determined woman who was our mother.

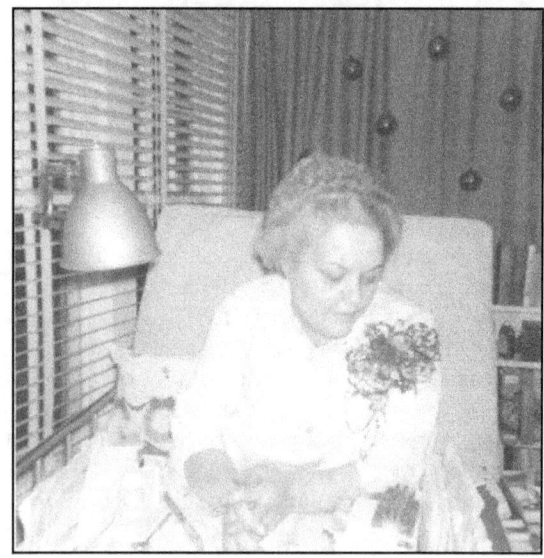

Rainie Clarke's Poetry

The following pages consist of four collections of Rainie Clarke's poetry written during the 1950s. In each case, these poems were written out longhand, revised and re-written, then (in most cases) typed into manuscript form. Rainie submitted many of these poems to *The Saturday Evening Post, Reader's Digest*, and other periodicals, but none was ever accepted for publication. She worked through an agent to try to find a venue for publishing her poetry, but was unsuccessful. She also corresponded with the popular poet, Ogden Nash, who was a major influence on her style and who encouraged her to continue trying. But for reasons that can only be dimly understood by authors, editors, and publishers, she was unsuccessful in convincing anyone to publish her poetry.

That really is a shame. Rainie's poetry is as diverse and deep as was her personality. It reflects her sense of humor, especially her love of nature, her romantic yearnings, her sympathetic understanding of the lonely and ageing, and her sardonic view of pretense and the often unpredictable absurdity of life. It was deeply informed by her life experiences, as all good poetry inevitably must be.

While her poetry is often wistful and often reminiscent of the sometimes melancholy verse of Edna St. Vincent Millay, another of her favorite poets and major influences on her work, it is never bitter or biting, never harsh or condemnatory, and certainly never self-pitying.

Reading Rainie's poems, one would never know that she had narrowly escaped death and fought her way back to functionality after being stricken down in her prime by polio, a disease that likely is unfamiliar to almost all of today's readers. Yet knowing her background of abandonment and adoption as a child, a young adulthood and early marriage of struggle to make ends meet, and a new mother whose normal life cut prematurely short by the cruelty of paralysis are crucial to understanding the depth of emotion, the hints of missed opportunities, the deep appreciation of the beauties of life, and the undercurrent of disdain for those who fail to try to make the best of whatever life has given them.

The poems of *Nest Feathers* especially display her wistful sense of the fickleness of fate and the foibles of humanity using

185

birds as their metaphor. Some show a strong influence of Ogden Nash, while others playfully demonstrate Rainie's broad learning and creative spirit.

Anno Dominates generally displays an entirely different tone. With affection and acute observation, Rainie examines the colors, flavors, and smells of the months and seasons, evoking the emotions of each with vivid imagery and an underlying linkage of the passage of the seasons to the stages of life. Although only in her late 30s and early 40s, Rainie shows a deep understanding and sympathy for the loneliness and internal life of the ageing.

New Leaves is the most diverse of the four collections, full of romantic yearnings and colorful imagery that hint at an inner life that never seems to have been exposed to others outside her poetry, a world of regrets, romantic yearnings for more than life can provide, and yet a steadfast optimism and self-confidence that all will be alright in the end.

Rigor Mortals pokes gentle fun at the pomposities and pretensions of human beings, from the housewife to the literary agent and from the road hog to the politician. Each in the end, gets his due.

And so, more than 50 years after Rainie wrote these charming, creative, emotive, and humorous poems, she too will get her due.

Nest Feathers

Rainie Clarke

FEATHER #1

My most carefully chosen plot
seldom thickens.
Many a rotten egg I've got,
counting chickens.

FEATHER #2

When I consider the untidy habits
of the feathered band,
I prefer observing two birds in the bush
to one in the hand.

FEATHER #3

And this is all I know of life
that shall convulse whatever Gods may be
with jollity and mirth;
always there lurks some force of gravity
to pull me down to earth.

FEATHER #4

I've watched the birds grow hungry. Frequently
they've died as winter comes.
I understand. I've often had to be
satisfied with crumbs.

FEATHER #5

Birds of a feather
flock together,
or so the saying goes.
But I'm wondering whether
they'd break their tether
if they suddenly changed their clothes.

FEATHER #6

She's sleek as an eagle,
her plumage is regal,
her costume's the very last word.
She's a sharp little dame,
but ain't it a shame?
She has only the brain of a bird.

FEATHER #7

I do not think the early bird
deserves a single kindly word.
His is a cowardly exhibition.
He's simply afraid of competition.

FEATHER #8

Point of comparison; figure of speech;
the Halcyon and I resemble each.
We nest on the crest of portentous waves
when we might stick tight to the beach.

FEATHER #9

The owl is a bird you'd best behoove.
To make an observation;
you can hoodwink the public if you've
an established reputation.

FEATHER #10

The Dodo was a stupid bird.
No bird more stupid than it.
What misdirected energy
to lay an egg of granite!

FEATHER #11

With fact that Nature frequently displays
a quiet sense of humor
who would quibble?
As when the peacock's footwear she surveys,
then shrugs her shoulders and says,
"Ishkibibble."

FEATHER #12

The sex life of the eagle
the timid has appalled.
If your sex life were airborne,
you, too, would soon be bald!

FEATHER #13
THE OSTRICH

She is unique; for her no succedaneum;
functional feet and vestigial wings.
If she insists on burying her cranium
at least she's keeping up her end of things.

FEATHER #14
THE PHOENIX

Begin again
where I began.
I'm
totalitarian.

FEATHER #15

I'd never be at a loss for words

if I owned a couple of Mynah birds.

(A shame this bird could not bestow its talent on the
minah poets.)

FEATHER #16

Bright flamingo in the sky
you are blushing! So would I
should I claim your family name,
you old Phoenicopteridae!

FEATHER #17

How lucky for the duck that he
is built so close twixt heel and knee,
for if he weren't, each time he'd kneel,
he'd drag an overbalanced keel.

FEATHER #18
HORSE FEATHERS

You may take your choice
by heck,
but as for me,
I'd rather be
a horse 's neck
in any class,
than be a horse's —
derriere,
so there!

FEATHER #19

Although he likes to parade his harem,
he's uninclined to want to share 'em.
Without his managerial talents
he fears the world might lose its balance,
and that is why
he blinks his eye
at each and every morning sky
and why he starts his A.M. mayhem,
and then expands his feathered vest
and gives a last triumphant shout,
because he knows without a doubt,
except for him, the sun would rest.
He struts in all his rooster beauty,
contented that he's done his best
to do his universal duty,
blissfully unaware his fate
will find him resting (fully dressed)
upon some sumptuous Sunday plate,
and that some other rooster's mayhem
will organize the Monday A.M.

FEATHER #20

The stork is smarter than you know.
He beats the owl for being wise
because he has arranged it so
you can't return his merchandise.

FEATHER #21

"The Stork's a myth," my son declares.
My son is half-past eight.
"He'd need a longer wingspread, Mom,
to carry all that weight!"

FEATHER #22
LA PALOMA PALAVER

As a harbinger of Peace
he's practically unemployed.
He's just about due for retirement.
Pity the void boid.

FEATHER #23
THE WOOD THRUSH

He sings the clearest morning call
and evening one, restraining lest
he burst the buttons on his vest,
a polka dotted tattersall.

Anno Dominates

Rainie Clarke

JUSTIFIABLE SUICIDE

If you shiver
in your cold rooms,
fighting off a case
of do1drums,
contemplating
hemlock berry,
don't be rash.
It's January.

SECOND SIGHT

The winter bough, though bent with ice,
is pregnant with a promised spring,
and winter winds both sigh and sing
of April.

Though resurrection waits for spring,
the seeds of it must germinate
in February to create
an April.

But February heaves a sigh
and slips away.
The time is late
and February cannot wait
for April.

Ah, there shall come a day when I,
with February, abdicate
because I have no time to wait
for April.

No single lifetime shall suffice

to savor miracles of spring,
so I shall be remembering
in April.

THE LIGHTER SIDE OF MARCH

Lamb and lion
are betraying
Nature's rule.
By Orion!
March is playing
April fool!

ABSENT APRIL

I take the days so carefully apart
and lay them neatly, one by one, aside,
dealing the year in small and separate piles,
stacking the months in groups. Now I divide
the year into its individual sections;
winter and fall and summer. Only spring
fails to remit her due amount of days.
May is amidst her fragrant floral maze.
June is residing where I last year left her.
April is absent; arrogant, errant April.
Like some precocious child who ran, because
she tore the pages of my memory,
April is absent.
What an empty year this one is going to be.

PANACEA

May may be a little slow
if you live at breakneck speed.
If you want your pace to grow,
maybe May is what you need.

JUNE GROOM

Bachelors betrothed in June are
struck with madness mildly lunar.
Rare the man remains immune
to Mendelssohn's immortal tune.

JULY

Sun tanned coats,
convention votes
and a bumper crop
of untamed oats.

AUGUST RAIN

Surely I shall love again
but never like this —
never with this wild, insane
fury of an August rain;
only like the gentle kiss
of early summer grain
as its tender tops barely miss
the train of my gown
on my barefooted way into town.
I shall never love like this
when I ever love again.
When I see the summer grain
laid to earth's barren breast
where my feet have pressed;
see it raped by August rain,
then I shall remember
famine in September,
and I shall be dressed
in the shadow of a frown
on my well-shod way back from town.

SEPTEMBER SMOKE

Your silver diadem of hair
is smoke from dying embers
left by the joy and the despair
of all your old Septembers.

WAITING

She stands beside her garden gate
wearing patience like a crown,
enveloped in the late
October gold and brown,
clipping the bayberries and bittersweet
and starting at echoes of an empty street.

NOVEMBER KNOCKS

November knocks.
I lean upon my rake
and watch the last remaining flocks
circle overhead, then dip their wings
and take their course toward softer climes.
My neighbors see me part the grass
and comb it neatly.
How could they guess?
It shall not easily be known
that only part of me collects
the leaves of last year's story,
and part of me has flown.

DECEMBER REMINISCENCE

When I am very old, they'll say
(and all the while with clucking tongue),
"She isn't quite herself today.
She thinks that she is young
again.   But strange!
The name she mentions is a name
she's never said before.
And why should such an old decrepit dame
prattle about magnolia blossoms
or pine trees, or white azaleas
growing near her door
where none have ever grown?
She spends too many hours alone.
And what a silly thing
for such an old, old lady to be mentioning
silver dust!
And more's the pity
that such a grandmama
should hum a half remembered ditty
in a cracked voice.   It's only noise."
But I shall smile

and busy gnarled fingers with
knitting one and purling one and dropping two,
the while amused
that bright young people such as these
should be confused,
could not observe the forest for the trees,
or they
would know that I am quite myself today.
Along with my Decembering,
I'm — sorting memories.

Rigor Mortals

Rainie Clarke

THE BIG SHOT

When they have flung the dirt
and placed the sod
and shed the public tear so bitterly,
figure the odds, my friend.
Let this be said of me,
"He's shot his wad!"

HAIL TO THE CHEF

When he arrives at Heaven's pearly portals,
before he tries his crown or tests a wing,
he'll swear to God by all his fellow mortals
the food could do with better seasoning.

THE ABSENT-MINDED LADY

She never felt much sillier
to her eternal shame.
The skeleton's familiar
but she can not place the frame.

THE POLITICIAN

Always to popular vote obedient,
observing majority rule as well,
he deemed it politically expedient
to make his eternal home in Hell.

THE YES-MAN

He more than willingly cooperated.
To this extremity ambition led;
when his dynamic boss expostulated,
"Drop Dead!"

THE AGENT

On facing his board of review
he nearly prompted Satan to repent,
when, giving the Devil his due,
insisted on retaining ten percent.

THE COMEDIAN

And this the only word that he
could say to his creator:
"A morbid thing occurred to me
on the way to this thee-ayter!"

THE HOUSEWIFE

She lent to life a charm and homely grace
with all the energy that she could muster.
They shrouded her in curtains made of lace,
and in her hand they placed a feather duster.

THE ROAD HOG

Up to and past the bitter end,
beyond his dying day,
he continued to contend
he had the right-of-way.

THE HAM

Deprived of an appreciative ear,
he grieved and died, unknown.
He finally grew too deaf to hear
his pear-shaped tone.

THE NEIGHBOR

They hold her funeral tomorrow.
Weapon: a Luger.
A thirteenth time she came to borrow
one cup of sugar.

THE FAT LADY

Though doctors continued to warn her,
a veteran calorie client,
they found the right thing to adorn her:
they purchased her shroud at Lane Bryant.

THE SOUTHERN GENTLEMAN

He bowed politely. Raised his glass to quaff.
His head grew thick the while his tongue grew
   thicker.
Upon his grave they carved this epitaph:
"A gentleman, suh, knows how to hold his
   liquor!"

THE TEXAN

Inheriting his final state of Glory
he'll shout with vigor;
regarding the celestial territory,
he knows, without a doubt, Texas is bigger.

THE REPORTER

The surest thing in life, he sneers,
is that it seldom varies.
His last by-line always appears
in the obituaries.

THE COMMUNIST

Here today and gone tomorrow,
Pravda stated.
He elicits little sorrow.
He deviated.

THE CRITIC

When his small soul effected its removal,
he felt disposed to issue his critique.
He'd not give the arrangements his approval.
He found the plot too weak.

New Leaves

Rainie Clarke

NEW LEAVES

New leaves
providing my parole,
whisperings, yea, louder than a shout
within my conscience,
God's intention
that I may yet have one more chance.
Resolutions should he made,
not in the cold and dead of winter,
but on the first appearance
of bright, tender, promising
new leaves.
They were designed that I,
an ardent lover
of world
and time
and space,
might turn them over.

AMEN

Spring is a tender love song.
Fall is a passionate cry.
Spring is a gentle beginning,
a tremulous start.
Fall is the last red
drop of experience
wrung from your heart.
I would not live spring over again,
although I may tend
to wish, fruitlessly,
that autumn might be
world without end.

I LOVE ALL THINGS IN AUTUMN

I love all things in autumn;
the haze upon the distant hills,
the mournful solitary trills
of birds that haven't quite the heart to leave;
that huddle on the barren branch
and barricade themselves against the chills
of winter's early preview.
All things in autumn please me;
the palette flash of pheasant cocks
along the edge of pasture;
acreage of shocks so vast
your eyes appear to be deceived;
the front yard maples
laying by their summer frocks
and laughing, though unleaved;
the mounds of russet, brown and gold;
more apples than the cider press can hold.
But of all things in autumn
I love best the perfume of the bonfires,
reducing to a residue of ashes, spring's desires,

and leaving me the warmth and glow
of things I know will last
through every icy blast.

THE COMPANY I KEEP

My dear, you must not stand and weep.
For I, who seem so much alone
discover that I shall be known
by the company I keep.
Here like a dusty chimney sweep
among the cobwebs, there invades
a company of lovely shades —
the company I keep.
Around, about my mind they creep,
products of memory and thought;
comparisons as could not be bought,
the company I keep.
So be it. Let the dreamer reap
associations from the past.
These are the friendships that shall last,
this company I keep.
And where the edge of endless sleep
shall lead me; here from There divide,
I shall admit with boundless pride
the company I keep.

IN THE MIDST OF MANY – NOTHING

In the midst of many – nothing.
In the midst of the mob, alone.
I am shaken by a rude
awakening in the multitude.
For all of the days of my life
I have stood a little apart.
He who has not known loneliness
amongst the throng
can never sing my song
nor hear the melancholy call
of isolation within the crowd
nor observe the loud
reverberations of a grieving heart.

DAYLIGHT SAVINGS TIME

That hour they robbed us of last spring
has haunted me the summer through
and all my plans for spending it
require at least a year or two.
Alas! I know myself too well,
and when November first comes creeping
through the window blinds, this year (at last)
it's ten-to-one I've spent it – sleeping!

BUT ONLY GODS

Thy glances pierce my heart and lay it bare.
They speak the thoughts withheld by thy sweet
    mouth.
A fluttering of wings departing south
on the last day of Autumn vintage air
stirs in my breast. Thine eyes have pinioned me
so that, like fair Dryope, I stand rooted to the
    ground.
I would that leaves and swiftly spreading bark of
    phantom tree,
obscuring all I know of life, save thee,
grew here, surrounding me.
Then might thou stand within my shadow
    murmuring sound
on sound of all sweet promises I fear
to listen of thee now.
So bathing in my shade and languishing
in perfume of my bough,
Thou'lt lean to carve they name upon my bark,
as thou hast carved thy image on my heart.

RETROSPECT

All the things I might have been
have gone dancing down the years
while bequeathing me a thin
heritage of tears.

All of those I might have loved
ever toward the past withdrew.
The rule, but one exception, proved;
Except for you, except for you.

DEBRIS

Never believe that I am bitter
over the likes of you!
But fractured heart makes a frightful litter.
See what you made me do?

TOUCHÉ

Call me a fool if it please you,
but let me make one thing clear.
Darling, it takes one to know one.
It takes one to know one, dear.

Whenever you're tempted to hand me
that shop-worn paternal smear,
Darling, it takes one to know one.
It takes one to know one, dear.

Put this in your pipe and smoke it
the next time you think I'm queer.
Darling, it takes one to know one.
It takes one to know one, dear.

SONNET FOR SUNBATHERS

The me who did not seek the shade
in time to ward off Nature's scathing
intolerance of tender maid
must now endure results of bathing
too often and too carelessly
outside society's sacred portals.
And now I hear cacophony
from all my fellow mortals
who raise the hue and shout the cry
and who exhibit righteous passion.
They're mortified that you or I
behave in such a fashion.
Ah, they shall never know the fun
of bathing naked in the sun!

BIRD IN THE HAND

Yesterday, I caught a singing thrush.
His silver-fluted call
echoed all desires that from my breast had ever
    sprung.
No bird had ever sung
such a wild sweet rapture.
I thought to place a band
to claim his capture
and then release him.
But I could not bear to part with him.
I held him to my heart and said, "Tomorrow,
I will let him go tomorrow."
Today I hold a dead bird in my hand.
I sample sorrow
but I do not understand.

WRITER'S CRAMP

While my heart rehearses
how to beat and bleed
and its rate reverses
back to normal speed,
I turn reason into rhyme
and I occupy my time
writing little verses
you shall never read.

LOST, STRAYED, OR...

I'm terribly absent minded
and five will get you ten
I'll never be able to find it.
Misplaced confidence again.

POINT OF VIEW

Let him who will, take the level road
with the graded leveled bed.
In the depths I can always secure my load
for the purple heights ahead.

SPRING FASHION

The Woods, a dowager queen in tattered lace,
white and once elegant, through which now shows
a patch of dull brown undergarments, grows
more restless daily, awaiting spring's young grace.
Winged creatures rearrange her shabby hair,
decorate her with ornaments of love.
Not to he outdone, moss's velvet glove
spreads soft new lingerie for her to wear.
Spring will arrive and bring her green brocade.
In its bouffant skirt purple violets
will peek from folds and, with the wearing, fade;
ferns hem her gown like oversized egrets.
All through the long, lush spring The Woods is so
like me, all dressed up and — no place to go.

REASONABLE FACSIMILE

"Whither goest thou, little maid,
in thy mother's shoes and hat?"
"I'm going a-milking, sir," she said.
Now what do you think of that?
She's returning the bottle to the store.
(Dressed to the teeth, like Mum.)
A bottle she's going to get two-cents for
to blow on bubble gum.

ASKANCE

What is it to me?
It is neither here nor there
whither you go
nor where you wander.
I am quite as free
as the suburban air.
It's only just by chance
that people see me stare
at the illusive yonder.

WOOLGATHERING

Give me a wide, a sparkling sky
and a mound of grass to lie on
and I shall spin such dreams as I
shall never dare to try on.
I shall weave upon the loom
of my imagination
a myriad colored costume,
a fanciful creation.
I'll trim it with an ermine cloud.
this robe shall have no seams in it,
and you may use it as a shroud
and bury all my dreams in it.

MULLED WINE

Where are you now?
Do you still enter that same room
with a new kitten's awkward grace,
illuminating any face,
causing the dull chintz draperies to bloom?
Do you still toss your radiant head
acknowledging some present "us"?
Beat slowly heart. 'Twas ever thus;
that time could stand so still
and yet two pair of eyes,
amidst a swarm of people,
meet and recognize
all that two souls may ever learn
for having lived one moment or an eon.
Where are you now?
And as for me,
how good (and dull)!
I hug the hearth; renounce the heath,
I toast my toes and bury
disturbing thoughts beneath
a glass of sherry.

And stammer little verses to assuage
the dulling pain of living out an age
of empty promises.
And I console myself
with time-worn sayings
and lying in my teeth!

CALENDAR FOR A SUMMER ROMANCE

Count on May for fruit and flower.

Count on June for wedding.

Count on Jan. and Feb. for tough sledding.

Trust April for sudden shower,

Nov. for table spreading,

Mar. to check where income's been heading.

Choose July for idle hour,

Dec. for decking hall,

Sept. and Oct. for fabulous fall,

but never count on August at all!

FARSIGHTED

Autumn is finger painting
in my woods again
and warning me that winter's ice and rain
shall quite erase
the brilliant complexion
of autumn's face,
and I must bear,
stark naked and alone,
the sight of unkempt hair
and frozen visage of that crone,
The Barren Queen of Bluster,
with all the power of will
that I can muster.
I'll grit my teeth and bear it,
show my mettle.
Eventually winter must soft-petal.

MARCH FOOL

Spring is impatient to be free
of winter's grasp.
Green stuff is sneaking furtively
along the cusp
of the brown hill. It seems to me
like will o' wisp
rising in marshland stealthily
from nature's clasp.
Now the last snow spreads disappointment
with its fall,
and the moist powder does anoint
the long brown hill,
while skeleton tree fingers point
me out the fool.
Snow covers every limb and joint,
obscuring all.

From winter's long confinement surely
March will redeem me.
March has delivered spring too early.
Spring is a "preemie".

MY CUP RUNNETH OVER

I sit so still and prim.
I card my wool
and darn my hose
and play Chopin and Mozart
on my spinet.
Up to its graceful rim
my cup is full,
and there are those
who'll never know that my heart
isn't in it.

PREROGATIVE

Now my passion has expired.
Now the inner spark has dwindled.
No more can it be rekindled.
When the sun was brightly fired
was the time for making hay.
Love and learn, I always say.

You may pay the fiddler for me
now the song and dance has ended.
Having Eros' charms offended,
now you do no more than bore me
with your foolish roundelay.
Love and learn, I always say.

La, sir! I'm a fool to listen
to the words I find so forceful.
You and Cupid are resourceful.
It need not be gold to glisten.
Silver tongues like yours may sway.
Love and learn, I always say!

BARE IN MIND

Bare in mind, initial introductions
or an evening's brief and shy encounter
or enthusiasm for a song,
generating memories sweet and strong.
Silent conversation that can bind,
Bare in mind.

Bear in mind the sight of lonesome litter
or the envied flight of brilliant plumage
or the sound of heels upon a floor —
unexpected vision at my door,
vanishing, tho' leaving me, I find,
Bare in mind.

Bear in mind a pleasant night of music
or the fun of sharing fresh baked cookies,
of a parting moment, all too brief,
climaxed with a verse on memo leaf,
to keep (unintended or designed?).
Bare in mind.

STORM WARNING

I shall forget. Ah, yes, there is no doubt of it.
And last year's story shall run true to form.
Still, I can say the best that I got out of it
was temporary refuge from the storm.

I shall forget. There isn't any question.
That others may avoid the web you spin
in future, may I make a small suggestion?
Bar your front gate and let no stranger in.

AN OUNCE OF PRECAUTION

Give thy shoes and gowns away
if thou'rt called upon to do so.
Give a winsome smile to suitor.
Stitch a seam and sew a trousseau.
Give thy hand, but play it smart.
Heed thy mother's warning, pray,
Save a fragment of thy heart
for a rainy day.

Now I mark the words my mother
spoke to me when I was young.
Now the deluge comes to smother
shrewdest words of mother tongue.
Wise am I and wise thou art,
if thou mindst what I say.
Save a fragment of thy heart
for a rainy day.

Let them tear thy heart to tatters.
Hang what's left upon thy sleeve.
All that ever really matters,

Daughter of rebellious Eve,
is to save a tiny part,
run amok or run astray,
but save a fragment of thy heart
for a rainy day.

HORTICULTURALIST

My thumbs are notoriously un-green.
I display no rapport with the ground.
But one bush I require in my garden
for the purpose of beating around.

HOUSING SHORTAGE

The Inn which once denied
admittance to the weary travelers
is still too crowded.
With all the knowledge
Man may yet attain,
he wallows in the penury of gain,
and all too often gain and gainful pride
are all that man has really deified.

UNACCUSTOMED AS YOU ARE

Speak your love when it blooms
ere the chance departs.
Lonely faces, empty rooms
are filled with tongue-tied hearts.